Other Books by Chamein Canton

Ms. Doesn't Stand for Multiple Sclerosis
Writers Club Press

You're Getting Married?
Writers Club Press

DOWN THAT AISLE
IN STYLE!

A Wedding Guide for Full-Figured Women

CHAMEIN CANTON

DOWN THAT AISLE
INSTYLE!

A Wedding Guide for Full-Figured Women

CHAMEIN CANTON

WindRiver Publishing • Silverton, Idaho

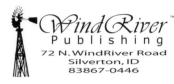

WindRiver Publishing
72 N. WindRiver Road
Silverton, ID
83867-0446

Queries, comments or correspondence concerning this work should be directed to the author and submitted to WindRiver Publishing at Authors@WindRiverPublishing.com. Information regarding this work or other works published by Wind-River Publishing, Inc., and instructions for submitting manuscripts for review for publication, can be found at http://www.WindRiverPublishing.com

Other fine books by WindRiver Publishing are available from your local bookstore, online, or direct from the publisher.

Down That Aisle in Style!
A Wedding Guide for Full-Figured Women

Cover Design by Cathi Stevenson
Book Cover Express
www.BookCoverExpress.com

**Cover photographs courtesy Alfred Angelo (left, center)
and David's Bridal (right)**
http://www.AlfredAngelo.com
http://www.DavidsBridal.com

Library of Congress Control Number: 2005935169
ISBN-13 978-1-886249-13-4
ISBN-10 1-886249-13-X

First Printing 2006
Printed in China

This book is dedicated to a group of the most amazing people I have ever known. They have unselfishly given me their unwavering support, regardless of the roads I chose to take in life, or my size while I traveled them.

Grandma Salley and Grandma Canton, Nana and Auntie Ruth, my dad Leonard Canton and my mother Mary Wallace. My sister Natalie Gordon and my brother-in-spirit, Joel Woodard. My twin uncles, Calvin and Cecil Canton, and Aunt Edna and Uncle Willis, who helped me bake my first wedding cake on an Easy Bake oven.

And a special dedication to my sons Sean and Scott, the two best sons in the world—may you choose companions in your life who meet the standards of your heart.

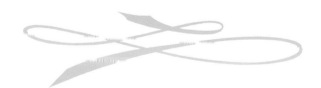

CONTENTS

TABLE OF CONTENTS

Foreword

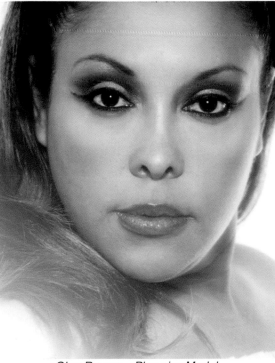

Olga Ramos – Plus-size Model

I was a very stubborn plus-size bride, determined to find my dream dress. But after many visits to bridal stores, I realized I was in trouble.

Not all stores carried plus sizes, and the few that did simply had large versions of gowns only small brides could wear. To make matters worse, I really wasn't used to wearing a dress at all. I finally hit upon the idea of trying on evening gowns, and I tried on every color and style.

I was trying to get the right fit and style for *me*. I wanted to be sure the length of the gown and the way the material wrapped around my body made me look good. I never quite found the perfect dress, but there were three gowns that I liked. So I wrote down what I liked about each one and went looking for a dressmaker.

My dressmaker considered my natural curves and used the information I'd gathered to help me flatter my features. My neck is long and my shoulders are nice, so we decided to show them off. She worked with me to create long hanging sleeves. The effect drew attention to my shoulders and made them say "Hey, Look at me!" I added a bit of lace to the mid-sleeve, but generally I stayed away from too much decoration. I felt it would only make me look bigger, and in my case less was better. The result was an absolutely gorgeous dress. It was romantic, elegant, and had just a hint of times past. It made me look and feel beautiful.

Life is too short to waste even one second on self-doubt. Full-figured women have been quiet and patient long enough—allowing smaller women to receive all the compliments. I will not give anyone the power to judge my smile, the sound of my laughter, or the way I choose to carry myself—because I am beautiful—and you are, too!

Olga Ramos

Inspiration

Melissa Stamper
Miss Plus America 1998
Executive Director, *Miss Plus America*

I was in pageants as a child. I had a great time because my mother and I would travel to different cities during the summer to compete. As much as anyone, I loved to compete and hated to lose. I loved dressing up and seeing a crown shine in the spotlight! *It was who I was.* So when I saw an advertisement for a plus pageant in Florida in 1998, I entered.

I did not expect to win. It had been years since I'd competed and walking onto a stage as a full-figured woman was nerve-wracking. But the memories of my childhood came flooding back and I chose to be proud of who I am. I won that national title, and due to my efforts during my reign, the plus division quadrupled in size the following year!

As a child I put my identity in my crowns. I felt they were proof that I was beautiful and confident. *But I've come to realize that my identity is my crown.*

Kathleen Bennett
Plus-size Model,
Miss Plus America's first cover girl, 2003

I'm surprised when people comment on my confidence. I'm dying to ask them, "Do you really believe I'm confident?"

My reaction comes from my childhood. When I was younger, I never listened to what I thought was baloney about loving myself for the way I was. I was too busy trying to be a size 7 to care about my own self-confidence. *I'm glad I finally listened.*

Nelle Gilbert
Plus Model

Celebrate your life, your commitment, and YOU! Embrace your womanly curves and prepare to embark on a new journey; a journey of LOVE. Being in love with my best friend has encouraged me to love myself, and each little dimple and curve. He's been my support, and loves to love real women with softness, curves, and confidence. I encourage you to embrace every laugh, every curve, ALL of you, and your love will continue to grow and blossom!

Valery Foley
Creator, *The Venus Divas*

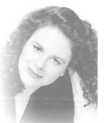

Who wrote the rule book that says we must base our self-worth on our size? Society? The media? Forget the rules! I say we should be healthy and find happiness at whatever size of beautiful you are. The world is passing you by while you sit around and lament your luscious curves. You want to be thinner? Drop the emotional baggage and you'll feel 100 pounds lighter!

Terreece Clarke
Plus Model

I never felt more beautiful than on my wedding day. Because the wedding was outside, I didn't put on my dress until I got to the park. There were no mirrors so I had to trust my bridesmaids that everything was in order. But inside. . . inside I felt so beautiful. One of my fondest memories, however, was when I stepped out of the car at the hotel. A girl stopped and said, "Look mommy, she's a princess!" It was the most magical day of my life.

Acknowledgments

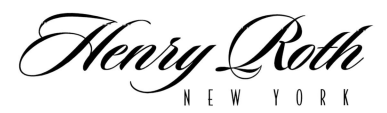

DESIGNERS

Alfred Angelo

1690 S Congress Ave Ste 120, Delray Beach, FL 33445 • (800) 528-3589 • info@alfredangelo.com
http://www.AlfredAngelo.com

Aurora D'Paradiso

The Formal Source • 11816 Race Track Road, Tampa, FL 33636 • formals@gls3c.com • www.formalsource.com

Cassandra Bromfield

400 West 42 Street, Ste 3C, New York, NY 10036 • (212) 502-5277 • cabcomp@aol.com • www.CassandraBromfield.com

Christopher Gambino

Gambino Jeans • 186 North Federal Hwy, Deerfield Beach , FL 33441 • (954) 425-8787 • info@gambinoapparel.com • www.GambinoApparel.com

DAVID'S BRIDAL

David's Bridal

(877)-923-BRIDE • http://www.DavidsBridal.com

DESIGNERS

Henry Roth
NEW YORK

Henry Roth

24 W 57th St, NY, NY 10019 • (212) 245-3390 • info@henryroth.com • http://www.HenryRoth.com

Mon Cheri Bridals

1018 Whitehead Road Extension, Trenton, NJ 08638 • custinfo@mcbridals.com • http://www.MonCheriBridal.com

Peggy Lutz Plus

7650 Bell Road, Windsor, CA 95492 • (707) 837-1897 • info@plus-size.com • http://www.Plus-Size.com

ROMONA KEVEZA
COLLECTION

Romona Keveza

450 7th Ave Ste 3105, NY, NY, 10123 • (212) 273-1113 • info@ramonakeveza.com • http://www.RamonaKeveza.com

DESIGNERS

Tasha Hill & Jeannie Ferguson

Big Girls United • 280 Herkimer Street Ste 6H, Brooklyn, NY 11216 • www.BigGirlsUnited.com

FLORIST

Wee Bee Country Florist

222 Broadway, Amityville, New York 11701 • (631) 264-0190 • (877) 264-0111 • www.myfsn.com/weebee

HAIR AND MAKEUP

Inner Beauty Consulting

108 McKinley Avenue, Brooklyn, NY 11208 • (347) 661-7703 • www.innerbeautyconsulting.com

Lisa Alpern

Lisafashionista • New York City • (917) 992-4559 • lisa@lisafashionista.com • http://www.LisaFashionista.com

Sittin Pretty Hair & Nail Solutions

194 A Broadway, Amityville, NY 11701 • (631) 264-7456

SpaIndex.Com

1511 M Sycamore Ste 104, Hercules, CA 94547 • www.SpaIndex.com

HAIR AND MAKEUP

Tanja Hrast

15370 Weddington Street Ste 118, Sherman Oaks, CA 91411 • (818) 692-9812 • info@tanjahrast.com • www.TanjaHrast.com

T.J. and Taschia

House of Essence • 525 Broadway Ave, New York NY, 11701

ILLUSTRATION

Nick Greenwood

mgreenwood@triad.rr.com

JEWELRY

Cynthia Sliwa

Apprecia Fine Jewelry • 1076 Monterey Boulevard, Hermosa Beach, Ca 90254 • (310) 980-8954 • appreciajewelry@aol.com • www.AppreciaFineJewelry.com

LIFESTYLE

Melissa Stamper

Coronet Productions • Miss Plus America Pageant • P. O. Box 4941, Monroe, LA 71203 • (318) 251-9711 • director@missplusamerica.com • www.coronetproductions.com • www.missplusamerica.com

Thea Politis

Elegant Plus • 180 Elm St Ste 1, Pittsfield MA, 01201 • www.ElegantPlus.com

ACKNOWLEDGMENTS

LIFESTYLE

Valery Foley (Founder) & Michele Weston

Venus Divas • www.venusdivas.com
Amaze Magazine • www.amazemagazine.com

Nelle Gilbert

Mo'Nique's Fat Chance 2006 Finalist
Call Me Curvy - Motivational • 785 Taneytown Road, Gettysburg, PA 17325 • www.CallMeCurvy.com

LINGERIE

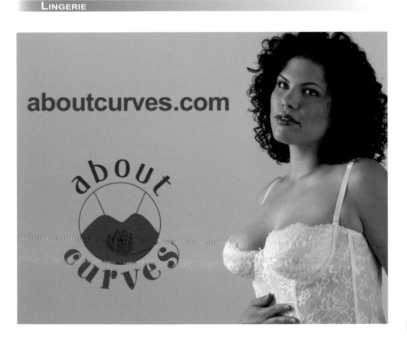

About Curves

7020 Greenbank Rd. Ste A, Baltimore, MD 21220-1111 • (877) 287-8963 • customercare@aboutcurves.com • http://www.AboutCurves.com

MASSAGE

Carol A. Canton

9926 Spring Lake, Clearmont FL, 34711

MODEL AGENT AND TRAINERS

Gwen Devoe

The Plus Academy • 244 Fifth Ave Ste 2373, New York, NY 10001 • (212) 561.0078 x1 • info@dseventsinc.com • www.dseventsinc.com

Irma Denson Skin Care

155 East 55th Street 4D, NY, NY 10022 • (212) 371-3413

Ja Tawn Avanti

Avanti & Associates Inc. • 205-18 112th Avenue Ste 201, St Albans, NY 11412

Rapunzel's Day Spa

106 Knapp Road, Lansdale, PA 19446 • (215) 368-7061 • rapunzelssalon@comcast.net • www.RapunzelsSalonAndSpa.com

MODELS

Cynthia Woodlief
Frances Brincat
Hansi Holloway
Jasmine Delgado
Joy Atkinson

DOWN THAT AISLE IN STYLE!

MODELS

Kathleen Bennett
Kelli Herbert
Lynette Schultz
Melissa Rios
Naiesha Brooks
Olga Ramos
Shanda LaRue
Stephanie Smith
Terreece Clarke
Tonya Jeter

PHOTOGRAPHERS

Brandyn Anderson

19763 Cranbrook Dr. Ste 116, Detroit MI 48221

Corwanda Black

Cordi Photography • 761 Marlborough,
Detroit, MI 48374

Christine Treager

1116 Aurora Drive, Pittsburgh, PA 15036 • (412) 512-
4591 • christine@treagerphotography.com •
www.treagerphotography.com

David Stith

328 N. High Street, Lancaster, OH 43130

Jake Mincey

Precise Creations

Jeffrey Fox

Second Floor • 25 Carrington Street, Lincoln, RI
02865 • (401) 729-1369

PHOTOGRAPHERS

Julia Bailer

216 Norland Avenue, New Orleans, LA 70131

Jun Pino

307 West 6th Street Ste 200, Royal, MI 48067

Oleg Vertiniskii

B#1 Photography • 474 48 ave, 26th Floor, LIC, NY
11109 • studio@1-b.com

Proline Studios

New York • (516) 775-4441 • ed@prolinestudios.com
• www.ProlineStudios.com

Zale Richard

3268 Motor Avenue, Los Angeles, CA 90034

RETAILERS AND SALONS

Angel Bridals

39 West Main Street, East Islip, NY 11730
• (631) 581-3330 • www.AngelBridals.com

Khris Cochran

Big Beautiful Brides • 180-A Villa Avenue, Los Gatos,
CA 95030 • (408) 757-2011

Plus Size Bridal

1029 Chapel Hill Rd., Burlington, NC 27215 • Fax
(336) 329-9025 • www.PlusSizeBridal.com

CHAMEIN CANTON

ACKNOWLEDGMENTS

RETAILERS AND SALONS

Sydneys Closet

11840 Dorsett Road, Maryland Heights, MO 63043 • (314) 344-5066 • (888) 479-3639 • www.SydneysCloset.com

WEDDING AND RECEPTION CENTERS

La Grange Inn

499 Montauk Highway, West Islip, New York 11795 • (631) 669-0765 • www.LaGrangeInn.com

Riviera at Massapequa

200 East Shore Drive, Massapequa, NY • (516) 541-5020 • www.rivieracaterer.com

The Wedding Center

3 Crooked Hill Road, Commack, New York 11725 • (631) 543-6898 • www.wc-commack.com

VEILS AND HEADPIECES

All You Need is Love

1193 Four Wynds Trail, Lexington, KY 40515 • (859) 533-1426 • polly@hatsandveils.net • http://www.HatsAndVeils.net

Veil Artistry

PO Box 340003, Columbus OH, 43235 • (614) 316-0839 • http://www.VeilArtistry.com

VEILS AND HEADPIECES

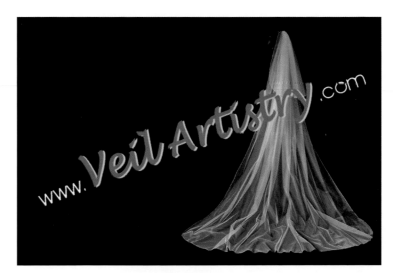

WEDDING CAKES

Micheline Cummings

Madame Butterfly Cakes • 22 Fireisland Ave, Babylon Village, NY 11702 • (631) 669-1069 • http://www.madamebutterflycakes.com

WEDDING EVENT PLANNER

Rosa Campbell

Event Planner

WEDDING INFORMATION

Wedding Sites and Services

P.O. 355, Smithtown, NY 11787 • www.weddingsitesandservices.com

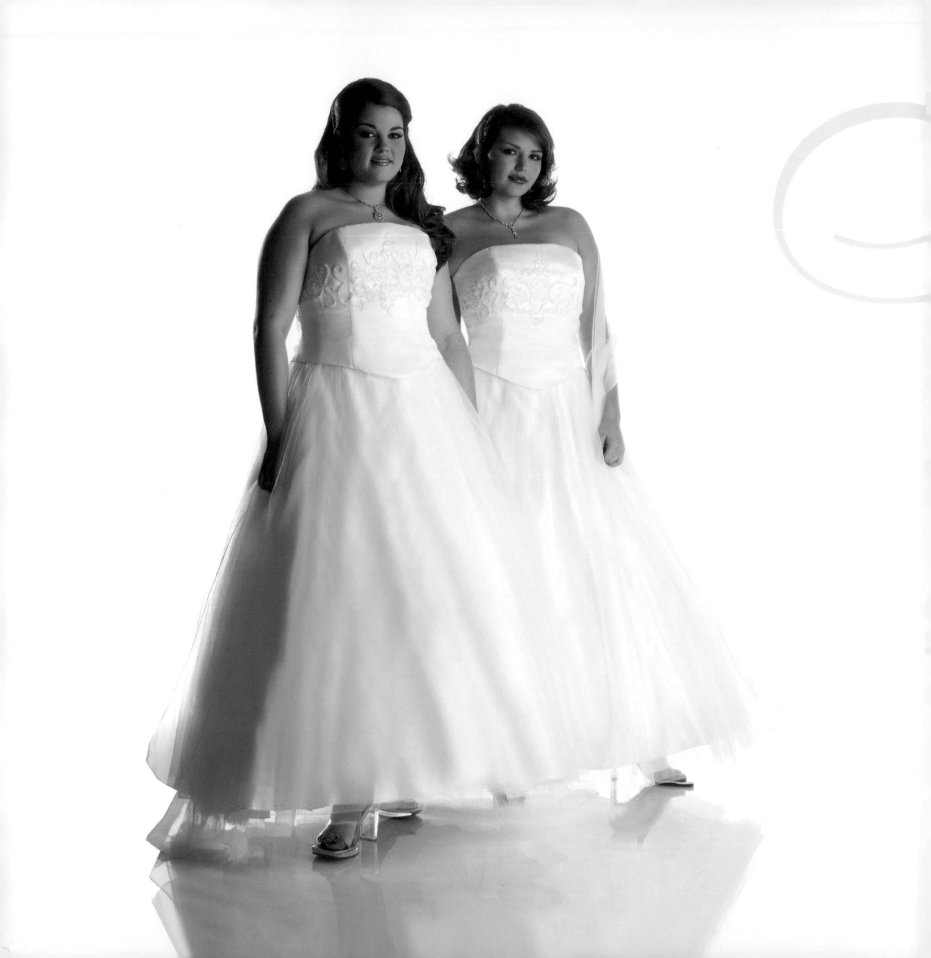

Hey You Beautiful Doll!

Before you begin shopping for your wedding dress—or any dress for that matter—there is one thing I want you to remember. Style is not about size; it's about attitude.

If you feel like a frump on the inside, I can guarantee you will look like a frump on the outside—no matter what you are wearing. On the other hand, if you feel beautiful on the inside, you will naturally project a beauty that is visible on the outside.

The brides and models in this book all have one thing in common, and it is not being full-figured—it's confidence! Their sense of self-worth lets them feel sexy and desirable, and there isn't a soul who can argue with that. As Miss Plus America 2003, Chenese Lewis, says, "Confidence shows when you walk into the room, remains as you exit, and is admired by all."

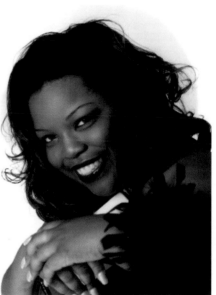

Chenese Lewis, Miss Plus America 2003

Full-figured women have made tremendous strides in front of the camera, in the glittering lights of Hollywood, and on the runway, but the most important stride any of us can make is in our own self-acceptance.

So, what does being a full-figured woman mean? Well, if you ask most people they will likely say it means you are fat or big with no distinction between either. Conversely, if you ask people what it means for a man to be big, you will hear answers like tall and muscular, even buff, before you hear the word fat.

The truth of the matter is, the phrase *full-figured* means much more than *weight*. Full-figured women come in all different shapes and sizes: we can be tall and leggy, or petite with delicate features, or have a muscular body that's built. In other words, we are not just round figures with legs; we have all kinds of curves with which to embrace life and the ones we love.

Look at it this way: the only actual difference between a size 4 and a size 14 is the *number*. Body shapes are universal and don't change by dress size. A pear-shaped size 6 will follow the same style guidelines when choosing a wedding gown as a pear-shaped size 18. There may be differences in the details, but the only substantial difference between the dresses is the size.

And while I'm on my soapbox, *full-figured* doesn't mean unhealthy or lazy any more than it means fat. For the last few years the focus of the media has been on weight rather than health—as if to say that all skinny people are healthy. Contrary to popular belief, size-four women don't fall into the stereotype of healthy and happy any more than full-figured women fall into the stereotype of sitting at home all day eating despondently. I'm all for losing weight to better your health, but if you're not happy with yourself, no amount of weight loss is going to help. Thin women may be in the media's spotlight, but *happy* women get more out of life, no matter what their figure may be.

Simply put, this is not an issue of them versus us. There are only women! And like all women, full-figured women deserve to be happy, to have confidence, to love and be loved by others, and to look absolutely *fabulous* on their wedding day! Every woman can look in the mirror and like *everything* she sees.

So get ready to learn how to bring out your own natural beauty, regardless of your shape or size, and have the time of your life doing it. Get ready to become the most beautiful bride your groom has ever seen!

Chamein Canton

Beautiful Clothing

The most important part of the wedding for many brides is the wedding gown. Your gown directly affects how you will look and how you will feel about yourself on your big day. Your gown should be an expression of your most confident and sensual self. The choices you make as you shop for your gown should be based on your own taste and preferences, and should be enhanced by some basic rules of style and design that show off your best features.

This chapter will help you learn what styles and fabrics work best for your individual body shape, how to get the best fit, and how to enhance the look with undergarments and accessories. It will help you choose the bridal salon that is right for you, and it will give you ideas on how to carry the concepts over to your daily wardrobe. (Remember, there will be a lot of tomorrows after the big wedding day.)

Before you begin, there are three things you should know:

First, despite the fact that 60% of all women fall into the full-figured category, you will likely be faced with some stereotypes when you go shopping for your gown. Be prepared for this, and don't let it diminish your self-esteem. You may find that sales clerks try to steer you toward certain styles. Don't let them. Demand to be shown the same beautiful gowns that someone who wears a size 10 would be shown. You may also discover a prevalent attitude in the bridal industry: that lots of detail will divert attention from larger sizes. Don't let yourself be led to gowns with a lot of sequins or embroidery work unless you prefer it. And if a bridal salon offers only a pat selection of gowns for "women," leave! There are other salons willing to accommodate your needs and preferences.

The second thing you should know is that when you walk into a bridal salon, your dress size *will* change—perhaps drastically. Please understand, this phenomenon is not a reflection of your figure; it does, in fact, happen across-the-board to women of all sizes. For example, women who wear a size 0-1 will usually wear a size 2 or even a size 4 bridal gown. Likewise, if you normally wear a size 16, you will probably need a size 18-20 gown. Why? All manufactured clothing varies, and wedding gowns specifically are sized to allow for alterations. Furthermore, they are based on size charts from the 1940s and 1950s. So don't let the jump in size scare you.

Third, you want to look for soft fabrics with enough give to flatter your figure. Stay away from stiff or shiny fabrics like taffeta as they tend to highlight problem areas you would rather camouflage. You want a fabric that flows with your curves rather than one that works against you. Some suggested fabrics are satin, organza, chiffon, stretch brocade, silk, rayon, soft linens, mesh lined with light lycra, silk velvet, silk or polyester georgette, jacquard, stretch brocade, and other soft fabrics.

Fortunately, there are things you can do to conquer the attitudes and quirks of the market. Begin with a confident attitude. Remember that you are, in fact, just as deserving of service and courtesy as any other customer. Then, take the time to be prepared. Use the following sections to determine what styles will make you look your best, and to learn the terms that you will be hearing at salons. Armed with knowledge and your beautiful, confident smile, you will be ready to work with people and find exactly what you want.

TABLES AND THE GLOSSARY

Tables are used throughout the book to show which clothing elements will work with your body. Elements that work well with your body are marked with a bullet (•). Dress elements that don't are left blank. Those that might work for you are shown with a question mark, often with additional details.

Also, I've chosen to focus on the fundamentals of fashion and style. As a result, some of the wonderful words that describe subtle differences in fashion design or the details of a design element have been placed in the glossary where you can quickly reference them.

THE PERFECT WOMAN

I've never met a perfect woman. Every woman is different, with her own perfections and flaws. The goal of this guide is to help women understand how a wedding gown can de-emphasize their flaws, emphasize their perfections, and affect the way people see them. However, to do that I need to first describe the *perfect* woman—lonely though she may be.

The perfect woman is 5'10" tall, weighs 120 pounds, has a perfect hourglass shape, and an oval face. The length of her arms and hands are such that the tips of her index fingers touch the curve of her hips at their widest point when they hang loose at her sides. Her neck gracefully raises her head above her shoulders to a height approximately equal to a third the breadth of her shoulders. The length of her legs is only slightly less than half her total height, and her thighs and calves taper smoothly from her hips to her ankles. Her feet are a size seven, and her bosom is a B or C cup. Her hairline exactly follows the curve of her forehead and probably falls past her shoulders in natural curls. *Believe it or not, there are gown styles this woman should not wear.*

Now let me tell you about real women:

- Every woman will be one of three basic body types: petite, average, or tall.
- Every woman will have one of six basic body shapes: inverted triangle, hourglass, rectangle, pear (triangle), round, or diamond.
- Every woman will have one of eight basic face shapes: oval, oblong, round, heart (or inverted triangle), square, rectangle, diamond, or triangle.

This translates into 144 unique combinations, not counting the impact of hairline, finger length, arm diameter, or the fact that ten hours on your feet will make your ankles swell—and not one single bit of this should stop you from looking wonderful when you walk down that aisle!

Now, as you consider what I have to say, remember that my recommendations are based on years of experience. Those same years have taught me that individual needs can vary. My goal is not to tell you hard and fast rules, but to help you better understand how clothing flatters a woman's body. Education is the key to success! So let's get to work, and since first things must be first, let's learn about our bodies.

BODY TYPES

The primary reason for knowing your body type is to understand how people will perceive your *height*. Your perceived height will determine how to manage the rest of your curves. It will also affect your skirt, veil, sleeve, and to a lesser extent, your headpiece choices. The basic heights used below do not take into account ethnic variations. For example, oriental people tend to be shorter than what I mention here. Determine which body type you have from the following definitions:

Petite   Petite women are shorter (5'4" and under), smaller boned, or clinically underweight when compared to the average woman.

Average   An average woman's weight is medically acceptable for her height of 5'4"-5'6", and her bone structure is statistically average compared to women around the country.

Tall   Tall women (5'7" and over) are often heavier boned when compared to the average woman.

BODY SHAPES

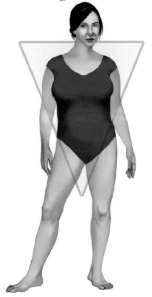

When it comes to looking your best, body shape is far more important than dress size. Your body shape is what determines which styles will look best on you: for example, which cut will make your waist look smaller, and which neckline will broaden your shoulders or minimize your bustline. The basic body shapes are:

Inverted Triangle   Full in the upper body, usually with broad shoulders. Hips are narrow and legs are usually long and shapely. Your gown should draw the eye away from your shoulders and focus it on your hips and legs.

Hourglass   The classic woman shape. Full bustline and hips with a narrow waist.

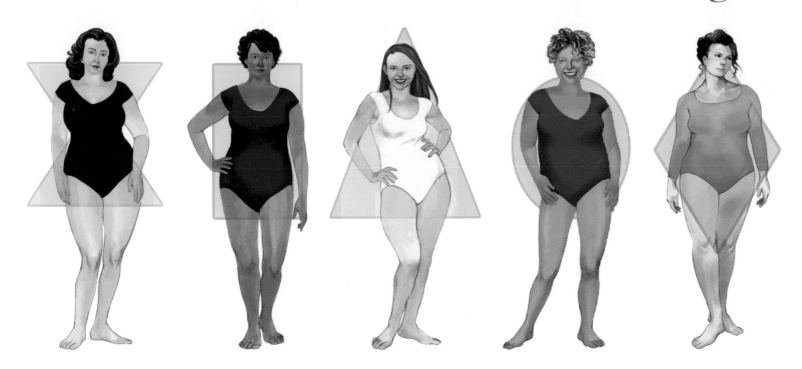

Legs taper to the ankle. Your gown should focus the eye on your waist and take advantage of your natural curves.

Rectangle   Sometimes referred to as a "boy" shape. Shoulders, bustline, waist, and hips, are equally wide. Your gown should draw the eye to your bustline and legs. The absence of visual interest around your waist will create the illusion of a narrower waist.

Pear /   Narrow shoulders and bustline with generous waist and hips. Your gown should draw atten-
Triangle   tion to your upper body, visually enlarging your shoulders to balance your hips.

Round   Average shoulders. Bustline and hips are equally wide while the waist is wider. Slender thighs and shapely legs. Your gown should focus attention on your neck and legs to increase your apparent height and elongate your upper torso.

Diamond   Narrow shoulders and small bustline, full waist and hips with legs that taper to the ankles. Your gown should hold the eye above your waist. This is most easily done by showcasing your bustline and broadening your shoulders.

If you are not sure what your body shape is, follow these steps:

1. Stand in front of a full-length mirror wearing only your bra and panties.

2. Face the mirror and allow your eye to follow the natural curves of your body. Look at your shoulders. Are they broader than your waist or narrower? Is your waistline well-defined or equal to your shoulders and hips?

CHAMEIN CANTON

3. Now look at your hips. Are they wider than your shoulders or narrower? Are your hips rounded, square, or straight?

4. Your legs are next. Are they long and thin? Are they shapely or muscular?

5. Now turn to the side. Are your arms thick and muscular, or thin? Are your breasts prominent, or do they align with your body? Keep in mind that large breasts can either protrude in front or widen to the sides. The latter is often the case in women with a wide back.

6. Check the motor in the back of your Honda. Is your bottom shapely and round, or is it smaller in proportion to the rest of your body? Is it close and high in relation to your back? Or does it slope a bit?

7. The final step is to use a handheld mirror and look at your reflection from the back. Is your back wide or narrow? Are your back muscles well-defined and toned? Where are your love handles? (And please, don't be offended. All of us have love handles!)

Now compare your results with the six shape categories and decide which most closely fits your figure. Once you have determined your body shape, you have won half the battle. You are now ready to consider styles that fit your particular shape.

CHOOSING THE RIGHT SILHOUETTE

Bridal gowns come in many different silhouettes. In the past, if you were "plus-sized" the selection was limited, to say the least. Fortunately, things are changing. Many designers are beginning to recognize that no two women are exactly alike—even if they wear the same size.

Alfred Angelo is an example of the many design houses that are providing options for full-figure fashion. Their bridal gown designs for full-figured brides are tasteful, lovely, and (dare I say it) more than a little sexy! They offer a wide choice of shapes and necklines to suit every body type. Still, while having options is good, keep in mind that some may not work to your advantage. Individual aspects of a gown, such as sleeves, necklines, or waistlines, can significantly change the appearance of your body—for better or for worse.

The following sections will teach you which styles will best enhance your body shape and minimize prob-

BODY SHAPES VS. SILHOUETTES

	A-Line	Ball	Column	Empire	Mermaid	Sheath
Inverted Triangle	●	●				
Hourglass	●	●	●	●	●	●
Rectangle	●	●		●	●	
Pear	●	●		●		
Round	●	●		●		
Diamond	●	●		●		

lem areas, and which styles you should avoid. The sections are organized to reflect the way most people see you. People naturally see the edges of an object before they see its details, so their first impression will be of your overall outline, or *silhouette.*

A bridal silhouette is the basic outline of the dress as a whole. Each silhouette represents a common combination of bodice, skirt, and sometimes neckline. It can be said that there are as many silhouettes as there are necklines, bodices, and skirts. However, there are six silhouettes that are so frequently used they form the foundation of gown design. They are A-line, ball, column, empire, mermaid, and sheath.

Rather than setting your heart on a particular dress you saw in a catalog, start with a silhouette that compliments your body shape, then work toward achieving the look and style you want through modifications to the neckline, waist, etc. If you do this, you will end up with a gown that takes advantage of all your beauty without compromising anything, and the gown will look as beautiful—or even more beautiful—than the gown you saw in the catalog.

Each of the six silhouettes depicted below represents a different way to accent the body, and each silhouette identifies the various body shapes it is best suited to and why.

A-Line Silhouette

A formfitting bodice flares out from the waistline to a full skirt, giving the silhouette its distinctive "A" shape. Today it is nearly indistinguishable from the princess silhouette. These gowns usually have a seamless waist. They balance the hips with the bust and often compensate for a minimal waistline. This is the most common of all the silhouettes, and it is good for all body shapes. For example, in the case of a rectangle shape, the A-line gently skims the body near the natural waistline to give the illusion of a defined waistline. On the other hand, if you have a thick waist or a bit of a tummy, the silhouette lightly skims the waist as it progressively flows to the skirt, thereby focusing the eye on the gown's flow rather than on your shape. Its wide skirt tends to reduce a taller woman's perceived height. However, when paired with a basque waist, it gives the illusion of height and elongates the torso on petite women.

Ball Silhouette

Also known as the traditional silhouette. This silhouette is characterized by a very full skirt that is fitted at the waist and flares to a formal length. The skirt waist is seamed at the natural waistline and can be of various styles. It features

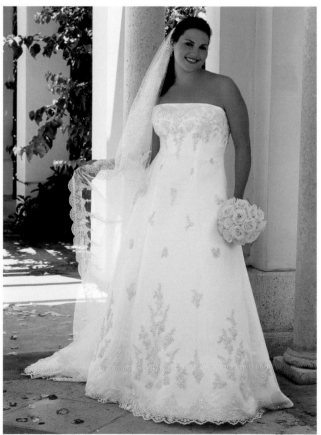

A-Line Silhouette

CHAMEIN CANTON

a formfitting bodice and a rounded, hoop-style skirt reminiscent of formal balls of the late 1800s. This silhouette balances the hips with the bust and is able to compensate for any differences between bustline, hips, or buttocks. It also compensates for a minimal waistline and is good for all body shapes, especially rectangle and pear shapes. The wide skirt tends to reduce perceived height.

Column Silhouette

Also known as the straight silhouette. This dress usually forms a straight line from shoulder to ankle that rarely, if ever, follows the curves of the body. It is generally recommended for women with an hourglass

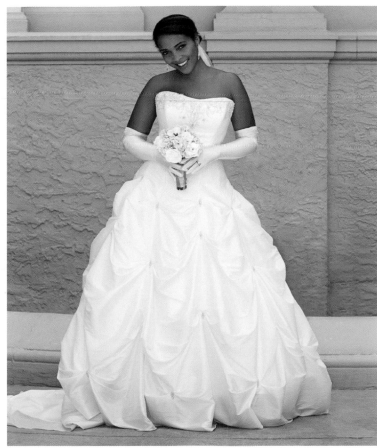

Ball Silhouette

shape. Any body area with a subdued curve will be lost in this silhouette. As a result, it emphasizes the differences between the upper and lower body, making them more pronounced. The narrow skirt tends to increase perceived height, making women appear taller. A fitted bodice with a straight skirt is also considered a column silhouette. A fuller variation of the column silhouette is the tank dress. It also falls in a straight line from the shoulder, but flares more at the hem. It produces a thinning effect on plus-size women which is further enhanced when combined with a bolero jacket or coat.

Empire Silhouette

A wedding gown that employs an empire waist (the waistline falls just beneath the bosom). The form is so distinctive that

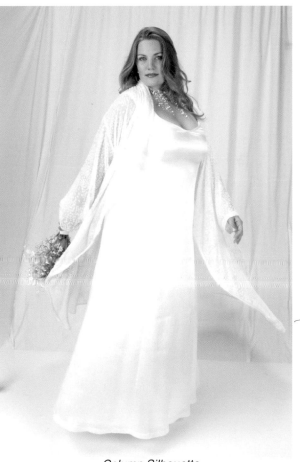

Column Silhouette

it earned its own name. This is the gown of choice if you want a nontraditional gown and don't have an hourglass body shape. It emphasizes the upper body, and will make women with large bosoms look very large. The narrow skirt tends to increase perceived height, making women appear taller. Peggy Lutz Plus produces a dress that fits like an empire style, but with "flattering, vertically curved seams" that end in a flared hem. They can be constructed with or without a train.

Mermaid Silhouette

This silhouette hugs the body until it reaches the knees or just above, then flares into a dramatic trumpet skirt. (Dresses made in this style are also known as fit-and-flare gowns.) The overall look is that of a mermaid with pronounced hips and fin-like tail. It is best suited for the hourglass body shape, but is usable by the rectangle shape if a waistline is designed into the gown. It emphasizes the bustline, knees, and hips. Women with broad shoulders should use a strapless bodice with this silhouette.

Sheath Silhouette

A formfitting version of the column silhouette. The sheath usually has a formfitting bodice accompanied by a straight or close-fitting skirt. The skirt is often ankle length, and sometimes has a slit in the front, side, or back to make walking easier. Gowns of this type often have detachable trains. It is perhaps the least forgiving of all the silhouettes. The closely fitted bodice and skirt will emphasize bustline, waist, hips, knees and ankles. It is only recommended for women with hourglass shapes.

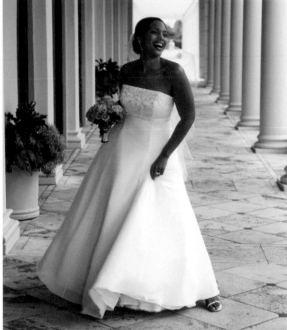

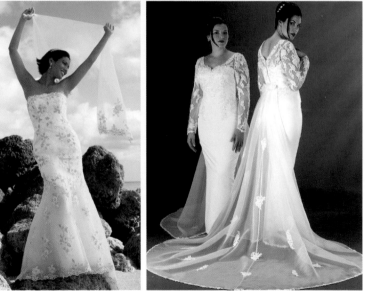

Empire (top), Mermaid (left), and Sheath (right) Silhouettes

CONSIDER YOUR FIGURE

One other concept may help you choose the right silhouette. The shape of a dress can either subdue or emphasize your figure. The ball and empire silhouettes subdue your figure by flattening lower body lines and curves. They produce a very traditional (vintage) bridal look and are good choices for brides that need to de-emphasize their waist, hips, or thighs.

The mermaid and sheath silhouettes will emphasize your lines and curves. They produce a modern bridal look and are good choices for brides who need to highlight their hips and bustline.

The A-line and column silhouettes are considered normal. They neither emphasize nor subdue your natural curves. These silhouettes produce the classic (stereotypical) bridal look. They should be used when a bride wants to show off the overall style of her gown rather than her figure.

NECK AND SHOULDERS

Once you have chosen the right silhouette for you, you can start filling in the details. Since most people will look at you from your head down, we will start at the top.

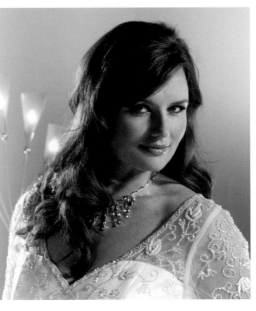

Neck and shoulder lines serve to frame the face and head and focus attention on the upper body. For instance, a woman with a large bust and broad shoulders may tend to buy V-neck shirts and sweaters since a V-neck draws attention away from the shoulder area and elongates the neck, making her appear taller. She also may be inclined to buy clothing with sleeves that are loose. (Unlike men, women tend to shy away from revealing the contour of their arms.) In cold climates, some women will layer a sweater over a V-neck shirt or buy a vertically ribbed turtleneck to lengthen and balance the upper body. (Me? I throw on a scarf over a good winter coat!)

On the other hand, a woman with narrow shoulders and broad hips will often choose high turtlenecks or a fitted blouse and sleeve. Why? On this woman, a V-neck would have the effect of drawing the eye down to the hips. Not a good thing.

So take a look in your closet and try on a few of your tops in front of a mirror. Do you see a recurring theme? Chances are you will, and that will provide you with the perfect blueprint to follow when shopping for the right neck and shoulder lines for your wedding gown. *Keep in mind that these lines will set the general style for the remainder of your gown.*

General Advice

The outline of your dress will define the overall "shape" people perceive when they look at you. This outline is generally defined by your gown's silhouette, but the details start with its neckline, sleeve type, and whether your dress has straps. The general shape and placement of the neckline, straps, and sleeves will control the flow of a person's eyes over your gown and dictate how they judge your appearance.

Placement

High necklines and full sleeves reduce apparent height and frame the face. Low necklines and hanging sleeves increase the appearance of height by lengthening the view of your neck and emphasizing your bosom. Longer or fuller sleeves will broaden the torso, balancing the hips. Short sleeves, narrow straps, or strapless gowns will narrow the appearance of your shoulders—unless you choose spaghetti straps. Their wide placement over the shoulders has a broadening effect.

Shape

The shape of a neckline draws the eye. Square and closed necklines will momentarily stop the eye, emphasizing your shoulders and bosom and subduing your hips, whereas scoop and V-shaped necklines speedily draw the eye down to a point and produce the opposite effect. Short and mid-length sleeves keep the eye on the upper body by drawing attention to the upper arm, while long sleeves and sleeveless gowns do not. Narrow straps subdue the upper body, causing the eye to move on. Wide straps draw attention to the upper body and significantly widen the perceived width of your shoulders.

As you consider which combination of neckline, straps, and sleeves to use, remember to consider your whole body. You want to draw attention to the shapely aspects of your body, and divert attention away from everything else. You can use all three elements of your gown to draw the eye, pause the eye, or speed the eye along. The use of illusion fabric can help moderate these effects. For example, if you have shapely breasts combined with a long neck, you will want to enhance your bustline to take focus away from the length of your neck. You can combine a sweetheart neckline with an illusion yoke and a choker to gain the shortening benefits of a wedding band neckline and the highlighting effects of a sweetheart neckline. However, before we go into more detail, I want you to become familiar with the following basic design elements:

Necklines

I'm sure you've already discovered that there are many different neckline styles with a wide variety of names. However, there are only four basic neckline styles: scoop, square, sweetheart, and V-shaped. There are three additional neckline styles that are so common, they deserve mentioning: the wedding band or high collar neckline, the jewel neckline, and the bateau neckline. These seven necklines will form the foundation of our discussion.

One more word about necklines. Their names and definitions frequently change according to geographical area and manufacturer. The Internet hasn't helped this problem since it has propagated incorrect definitions through mislabeled images or simple misunderstandings. If you understand the basic neckline styles, however, you will recognize them no matter what names they are given.

Following are neckline descriptions in order of how people normally observe you—from the top down. If more than one neckline is good for your shape, then choose between them to create the style you prefer.

Wedding Band Neckline

This is a formal, very high collar that fits snugly around the middle of the neck and just brushes the chin in a choker effect. It can be ornate or plain, and frequently tops a lace or net overlay that reveals portions of the upper chest. It is also known as a high collar neckline. This neckline reduces height and dramatically frames the face. It subdues the bosom in favor of the face, but has the effect of broadening the shoulders, especially when lace or net inserts are not used to enhance the effect of a full cloth yoke.

A common version of the wedding band is the elegant Queen Anne neckline. It cups the back of the neck with a choker effect, but leaves the front of the neck completely exposed. The Queen Anne is usually combined with a sweetheart neckline, but can be combined with others.

An uncommon version of this neckline is known as the Queen Elizabeth neckline. It has a collar that is very high and often flared in back, sloping gently and becoming narrower as it circles the neck to the front, ending in a "V," square, or sweetheart neckline.

A plain, high collar neckline with a notched-V in front is commonly referred to as a mandarin collar.

Associated Necklines

Wedding Band	Queen Anne
High Collar	Mandarin
Queen Elizabeth	

NECKLINES VS. BODY SHAPES

Specialty necklines are listed here only if they differ appreciably from their basic neckline.

	Inverted Triangle	Hourglass	Rectangle	Pear	Round	Diamond
Wedding Band		●	●	●		
Jewel		●	*	●		●
Bateau		●		●		●
Sabrina		●		●		●
Scoop	●	●	●	●	●	●
Square		●		●	●	●
Sweetheart	● †	●		● ‡		
V-Neck	●	●	●	●	●	●
Contessa		●	●	●	●	
Fichu		●	●	●	●	●
Portrait		●	●	●	●	●

*   *If combined with an A-line silhouette.*
†   *If combined with a strapless gown.*
‡   *If combined with a hanging sleeve or a portrait collar.*

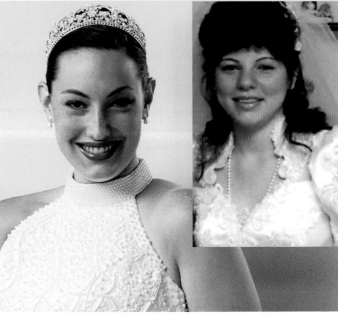

The Wedding Band and Queen Anne necklines

Jewel Neckline

This is a round neckline that follows the base of the neck. It reduces height, but does not frame the face. It is a good style for smaller bustlines since it makes them look larger. It is an especially attractive neckline on sleeveless gowns, and is excellent for tall women with broad, shapely shoulders.

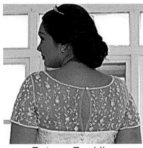

Bateau Neckline

The upper edge of this neckline follows just below the line of the collarbone and runs across the front and back, meeting at the shoulders. This style has little effect on height, but highlights a shapely neck and slender shoulders. It also makes a small bust look larger.

Bateau Backline

A version of the bateau known as the Sabrina neckline runs slightly higher than the standard bateau, along (rather than below) the collarbone.

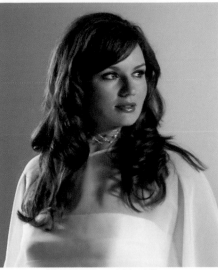

Illusion Jewel Neckline

Associated Necklines

Jewel	Scoop
Bateau	U-Neck
Sabrina	

Scoop Neckline

The basic scoop is one of the most common necklines. The upper edge of the neckline rests above the bosom in a "U" shape. It increases height and gently highlights cleavage. This neckline is a good choice for women with average breasts who want to include straps or sleeves to broaden narrow shoulders.

The deep U-shaped scoop neckline rests low over the bosoms (see décolletage) and is a good choice for women with larger breasts and narrow shoulders who want to draw attention away from the face and neck.

Square Neckline

The basic square neckline is also

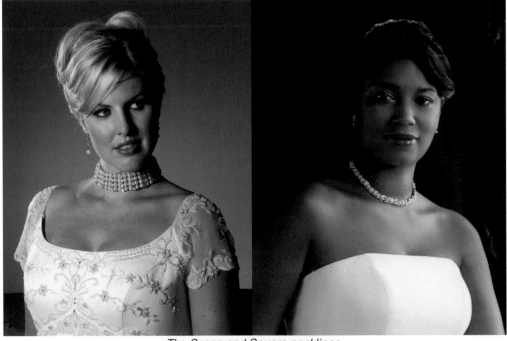

The Scoop and Square necklines

a very common neckline. It is frequently used with sleeveless and strapless dresses. Its upper edge rests above the bosom in a square shape. Its effect is to increase height and subdue the waist and hips (remember that a straight line will stop the eye), but it does not highlight cleavage. The square neckline is a good choice for women with average breasts and broad shoulders, especially when used without sleeves or straps. Women with overly large breasts can use the square neckline to take advantage of their bosom without drawing too much attention.

The court neckline is created by lowering the square neckline over the breasts to expose cleavage. This increases the sensuality of the gown without losing its elegant, traditional lines.

The contessa neckline is created by combining a square neckline with a strapless bodice and short hanging sleeves (often in a puffed style). The sleeves may or may not be attached to the gown itself, but the neckline and sleeves form a continuous line across the arms and chest when the arms are resting at the sides of the body. This neckline widens the torso without broadening the shoulders, and is a good choice for women with broad shoulders, small breasts, and a narrow waist.

Sweetheart Neckline

The upper edge of the sweetheart neckline cups the top of the breasts to form the upper half of a classic heart shape. It increases height and highlights the shape of the breasts. It is a good choice for women with broad shoulders and shapely breasts. It should not be used by women with overly large breasts unless they specifically want a décolletage look.

V-Neck Neckline

The upper edge of the V-neck neckline rests above the bosom in a "V" shape. It increases height and highlights both breast shape and cleavage. It also has the effect of moving the eye rapidly over the breasts toward the waist and hips. It is a good choice for women who want to emphasize their bosom without subduing their waist or hips.

Associated Necklines

V-Neck   Décolletage
Halter

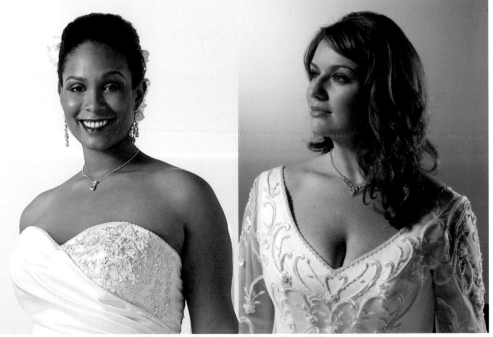

The Sweetheart and V-neck necklines

The halter neckline is created by combining the V-neck neckline with a halter strap of any kind and no sleeves. It has a more daring look, and is good for emphasizing shapely necks and bosoms while subduing the shoulders. It draws the eye down in a narrow path from head to waist.

A very daring décolletage neckline is created when the V-neck neckline rests low over the bosom. This neckline should generally be avoided unless you have a very shapely upper body and narrow waist.

Neckline Attributes

Neckline attributes are common enhancements that emphasize or soften the effects of a gown's basic neckline. They are often referred to as necklines, although this is not accurate. They are merely modifications of the basic necklines.

A *notched-V* neckline is any neckline that includes a V-shaped notch over the cleavage. It is most frequently combined with a square neckline as a means of highlighting cleavage. Adding a notched-V to a neckline will cause the eye to return to the center of the body, subduing the shoulders and upper torso.

A *keyhole* neckline is created by combining any neckline with an oval or teardrop opening at the base of the neckline. It is more dramatic than the notched-V, but serves the same purpose.

A *décolletage* neckline is any plunging neckline that generously reveals the bosom. The most common décolletage necklines are the deep U-shaped neckline and the plunging V-neck neckline, but it can also be created using other necklines, usually by adding a notched-V or keyhole to the neckline. It's worth noting that the décolletage neckline can *stop* the eye. If you don't believe me, remember Jennifer Lopez's Versace dress at the 2000 Grammy Awards? No one remembers how the bottom of the dress looked. Décolletage necklines are showy, but if you prefer men looking into your eyes when they talk to you, do not use this neckline.

A *scalloped* neckline describes any neckline that has a scalloped edge around the front half or the entire neckline. A sweetheart neckline (especially if the cups over the breasts are small or shallow) is often confused with a scalloped neckline because of the small curvature of the cut. Scalloping softens the design of a neckline, causing the eye to speed over its edges.

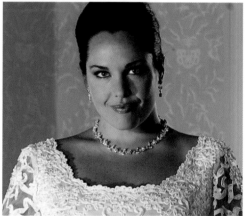
Scalloped Square Neckline

A *portrait* neckline is any neckline with an added broad collar. The collar can be created in many ways, including the addition of heavy lace or contrasting fabric. The most common form of a portrait neckline is a collared scoop neckline. The portrait neckline heavily frames the head and face and stops the downward descent of the eye. It is a good choice for women with shapely shoulders or necks.

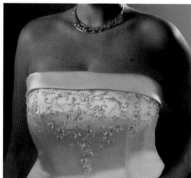
Portraited Square Neckline

A *fichu* neckline is any neckline with an added shawl or similarly folded or gathered cloth tucked into the neckline or tied over the bosom. The effect adds significant bulk to the upper body and is a good way for pear-shaped women to balance their hips with their shoulders. The most common form of the fichu neckline is a V-neck neckline with a shawl around the neck that is tucked in at the cleavage. This neckline has a very Victorian look.

Compound Necklines

There are six common neckline terms that are defined by a combination of strap, neckline, bodice, or sleeve styles

Asymmetric The left side of the upper torso exhibits sleeve, strap, neckline, or bodice attributes that are not used on the right side of the upper torso, or vice-versa.

Ballerina Any sleeveless bodice with spaghetti straps.

Contessa Any neckline (usually a square neckline) combined with a strapless bodice and short, hanging sleeves. The top edge of the sleeves are usually at the same height as the neckline, forming a continuous line across arms and torso.

Halter Any neckline combined with a sleeveless bodice and a neck halter.

Off-the-Shoulder Any strapless bodice that includes hanging sleeves.

Strapless Any neckline that is not combined with straps or sleeves (a dropped sleeve is the exception).

Illusion and Necklines

Illusion is a fine, semi-transparent netting or tulle used for both wedding gowns and veils. When used with a gown, it will show the shape of the body without losing the effect of the cloth it accompanies. It works best when used to replace a piece of cloth on your gown in order to highlight a point of interest or to create the effect of two necklines. For example, a woman with a generous bosom and narrow shoulders would normally choose a wedding band neckline with covered shoulders and elbow- or full-length sleeves to broaden her upper body shape, but she could also choose a sweetheart neckline to show off her natural curves and use illusion to simulate the wedding band neckline in order to widen her torso. A common example of this use of illusion is the Queen Anne neckline with an illusion yoke and full sleeves. Thus, the full effect of the cloth is present while still highlighting her curves.

Illusion can also be used in the opposite sense to add cloth where normally none would be used. The effect in this case is not as good as substituting cloth with illusion, but it is still quite valuable. For

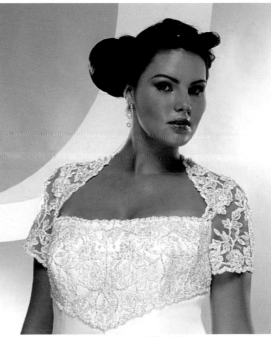

Illusion Jewel Backline

NECK AND SHOULDERS

example, a woman with broad shoulders and short arms would normally use a strapless, sleeveless dress to narrow her body shape, but she also needs to clothe her arms to give them a greater sense of length. The compromise is to use an illusion sleeve or a short bolero jacket made of illusion to add length to the arms while still moderating the breadth of her shoulders.

Choose the neck and shoulder lines you need to suit your body's shape, and if they prove to contradict other elements of your gown, use illusion to produce the compromise.

Shoulder Lines

Your shoulder line controls the breadth of your upper body. The eye sees the dress before the skin, so a strapless dress has the effect of reducing the breadth of your shoulders, while a strapped or sleeved dress will broaden your shoulders.

Shoulder lines are defined using *straps*. Straps are not sleeves. You can have a strapless dress with sleeves (the contessa neckline is one such example) or a sleeveless dress with straps (a halter neckline).

It's important to remember that I'm using the word *strap* to describe cloth of any width that covers part or all of the shoulders.

The illustrations below depict the different kinds of straps and how they affect body shape. The list starts with the thinnest straps first to the thickest straps last.

STRAPS VS. BODY SHAPES

	Inverted Triangle	Hourglass	Rectangle	Pear	Round	Diamond
Strapless	•	•	?*	•	•*	
Spaghetti Straps		•		•	?‡	•
Straight Halter		•	•	•	?‡	†
Crossed Halter		•	•	•	?‡	†
Neck Halter		•	•	•	?‡	
Full Yoke		•	?*	•		•

* Depends on the gown silhouette.

† If shoulders are very narrow, halter will work against you.

‡ If upper body area is somewhat more rounded, the straps can appear to pull or dig into skin. Test the look thoroughly from all sides before making a choice.

Spaghetti Straps

Very thin straps worn directly over the collarbone. Spaghetti straps are a specific kind of straight halter. Because of their wide placement on a gown, they make broad shoulders look wider, an exception to the effect generated by other straps. They add width to smaller upper bodies and balance the shoulders. If a corseted bodice is not used, the overall dress weight should be light (spaghetti straps don't have a lot of strength; they would cut into your shoulders if they did).

Straight Halter

A strap of any width usually worn over the collarbone, but it can be worn on the shoulder. When attached in front over the bosom and combined with the V-neck neckline, it creates the classic halter neckline. It generally has a neutral effect on shoulder width, but increasingly broadens the shoulders as strap width increases. Any bodice type can be used because halters can bear much more weight than spaghetti straps, but there are still limits.

Cross Halter

A strap of any width usually worn over the collarbone, but crossed over before attaching to the neckline. It slightly broadens the shoulders, with an increasing effect as the strap width increases. It can bear moderate dress weight.

Neck Halter

A strap of any width attached in front above or beside the bosom, and crossing behind the neck rather than attaching at the rear neckline. It slightly reduces shoulder breadth, with a decreasing effect as strap width increases. It can bear moderate dress weight.

Full Yoke

The widest of the straps, fully covering the shoulders. It broadens the perceived width of the shoulders to their widest, and can bear the most dress weight.

Attachments

Straps can be attached to the bodice in a variety of ways. The traditional method is to attach them on the front neckline beside or above the bosom, and on the back neckline at approximately the same points. However, straps can also be attached at a single point midway along either the front or the back neckline, or anywhere in between. Straps can also be attached wide of the bosom, right up to the underarm area (al-

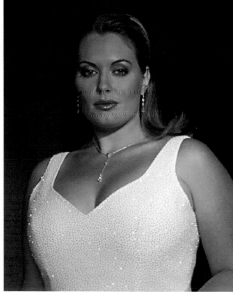
Straight Halter

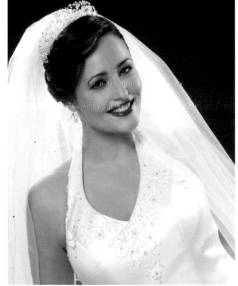
Neck Halter

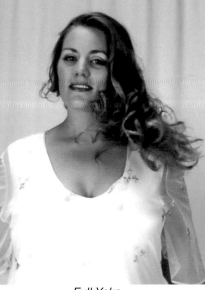
Full Yoke

though dress stability requires the opposite ends of straps connected in this manner to fasten at a point in the center back or to cross in back and fasten on opposite sides).

Straps can also be reversed front-to-back. For example, a crossed-and-straight halter combination can be worn with the cross in front or in back.

Dress weight is a significant consideration when selecting your strap solution. A dress with a long train or a ball gown with layers of satin fabric might find itself on the floor several feet behind you if you choose a strapless dress. There are three things that can hold a dress in place: straps, your bosom, and the bodice via friction against the sides of your body. Friction doesn't count for much when smooth fabrics like silk or satin are involved, and if you happen to have a small bosom, then something will have to give—either you'll need wide straps or a light dress.

YOUR BACK

As we discuss your wedding gown, we'll put a lot of effort into the front—after all, that's where most of the action is! However, during your wedding ceremony your guests will be looking at your back. How your back is perceived depends on your neckline and veil. We'll discuss your veil later; for now, let's talk about that neckline.

Most of the rules governing the front neckline apply to the back neckline as well. You obviously won't need to worry about your bosom, but you will need to worry about your shoulder blades, neck, and spine. Get someone to take a photo of you in a backless dress. Better still, have your mother, sister, or a good friend take a picture of your back with no clothes on. This will help you see what you're working with.

You will need to worry about how the flesh folds around your underarms when your arms are at your sides (important for strapless dresses). You should also consider where the line of your bra falls. Ladies with cup sizes D through E should be extra careful

BACK NECKLINES VS. BODY SHAPES

	Inverted Triangle	Hourglass	Rectangle	Pear	Round	Diamond
Wedding Band		• *		•		• †
Jewel		•	•	•		•
Bateau		• *	•	•		•
Scoop	•	•	•		•	•
Square	•	•	•	•	•	•
V-Neck		•	•	•	•	•
Décolletage‡		•	•			
Portrait/Fichu		•	•	•		
Asymmetric		•	•	•		•

* A large bosom will cause this neckline to pull in the back.

† A wedding band neckline would slim the upper body nicely; however, one must balance the look with either an A-line skirt, corseted bodice, or fitted bodice.

‡ When used on the back of the gown, the décolletage neckline usually describes a backless gown.

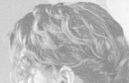

that their wider halters and straps are not showing, and that the fit is flush and not tight against their skin to help avoid the dreaded bra overhang.

Custom dresses can generally have any neckline on the back or front. The exceptions are the collared necklines (wedding band, portrait, and fichu) where the back neckline is defined by the front neckline, and the sweetheart neckline, which simply doesn't make sense on the back. Stock dresses will either match the necklines front-to-back, or use a subdued form of the front neckline on the back.

As a general rule, the various body shapes have the following back attributes:

Inverted Triangle	This body shape has a wide back and broad shoulders that are often well-defined due to a larger bone structure.
Hourglass	This body shape has an average back and shoulders that are usually fleshy or muscular.
Rectangle	This body shape has a slim back and shoulders. The back can appear muscular and/or slim.
Pear	Small shoulders and back define this body shape.
Round	An average back and shoulders define this body shape, but the back is usually broad and round.
Diamond	This body shape has a narrow upper and lower back, with a wider mid-point, and shoulders that usually appear slim or even bony.

Finally, a word about straps and your back. With the exception of halter straps, you will generally be forced to use the same straps on your back that you have on your front. Only custom dresses will change this. Strapless dresses can be the least forgiving if they don't fit properly. You may look fabulous in front, but have pinched skin around your underarms and along the neckline in back, forcing you to use a shawl or the veil to hide the imperfections. To avoid this, make sure the dress fits snugly enough to avoid your cups running over, and loose enough so that you can breathe freely.

Halters give you some options. A crossed halter will hide an imperfect back without significantly broadening the view of your shoulders, and a neck halter will give the back the same effect as a strapless gown. If you have decided to use a halter in front, use the halter in back to your best advantage—and remember that few (if any) of your wedding pictures will include your back.

BODICES

The word *bodice* means two things. First, it describes the upper-half of a gown. Second, it refers to the midsection of the upper gown—the area that isn't a sleeve, cuff, neckline, shoulder line, or waist. The bodice, therefore, is very important. It is the *frame* of the dress.

In construction terms, the foundation is the most important part of a building, with the frame running a close second. When an architect designs a home, he provides the builder with details for constructing the framework of the house. So in essence, the *frame* is the basis for the overall look the home will have once it's completed. While architects design homes for individual clients using a blueprint to convey their construction designs, bridal gown manufacturers design gowns using a combination of current trends, body shapes, and body types as their blueprint. Your body shape and type automatically provide them with a *foundation* on which to build.

Now, you might begin to panic since bodices and waistlines deal with an area most women (all shapes and sizes included) are inherently self-conscious about, *their tummies*. But as with many other aspects of fashion, it's an area we address in our everyday lives—whether we're aware of it or not. I'll use my own body as an example. I basically have an hourglass shape; however, I do have a tummy. So let's say I'm in the market for a pair of slacks. I automatically discount those with pleats since they tend to highlight the stomach. Instead, I look for slacks with a flat front. I also stay away from pleated skirts or dresses where fabric gathers around my midsection. On the other hand, if I were a pear shape I would look for A-line skirts that define my waist while de-emphasizing my lower body. The same principle applies to bodices.

There are only three types of bodices in the world: *corseted*, *fitted*, and *blouson*. You can decorate these bodice types in many different ways, but there are only the three.

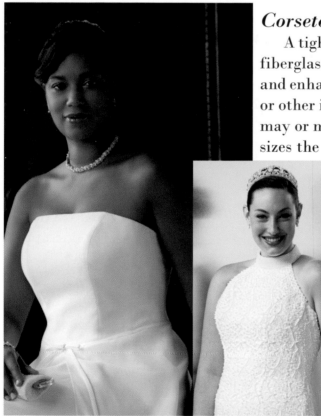

Corseted and Fitted Bodices

Corseted Bodice

A tight fitting bodice that uses tensioned material, including leather, fiberglass, and nylon elastic (originally whale bone), to shape the body and enhance the waistline. Corseted bodices that use fiberglass, wood, or other inserts to force a shape are said to be *boned*. Corseted bodices may or may not include lacing or hooks up the back or front. Emphasizes the waist, creating a waistline if needed. Tends to draw the eye up—not down—which broadens the perceived width of the shoulders. Best used with sleeveless or, better yet, strapless gowns. A corseted bodice should be avoided by inverted triangle and well-endowed hourglass body shapes unless the gown is strapless.

Fitted Bodice

A form-fitting bodice that is never strapless. It is fitted close to the body with vertical darts or seams in the front and up the curved lines of the back. It can be used with a full range of necklines and straps.

Note that the cut of the bodice will be determined

by a combination of body shape, style, and the silhouette. A bodice should not be cut too loosely when accommodating body shape. In fact, these adjustments should be quite small.

Blouson Bodice

A loosely fitting bodice that is not cut to fit the shape of the body. The traditional blouson bodice has a drooping fullness in its fabric that blouses over a gathered waist. It balances the midsection with the hips, minimizing the waistline. A blouson bodice should be avoided by round and diamond body shapes.

Specialty Bodices

There are two specialty bodices: the ballerina bodice and the empire bodice. These are not true bodices in the sense that they define the midsection of the body or connect the neckline with the waistline. These bodices are actually a combination of bodice, neckline, and straps.

The *ballerina bodice* is a combination of a blouson bodice, a scoop neckline, and spaghetti straps. It works well with those body shapes that are naturally complimented by the spaghetti straps: hourglass, pear, and diamond. It should be avoided by the other body shapes where the straps can cut across the shoulder or make the shoulders appear broad or bony.

Empire bodice is an infrequently used term for a dress with an empire waistline. Generally, the terms *empire bodice, empire waist,* and *empire silhouette* all describe the same dress. However, it is best to avoid using the phrases *empire bodice* and *empire silhouette*. Instead, select a silhouette that accurately reflects the skirt (such as the A-line or sheath silhouettes) then use the term *empire waist* to describe the waistline.

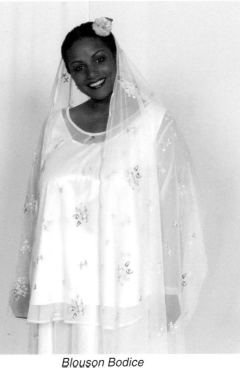

Blouson Bodice

WAISTLINES

Waistlines are an intrinsic part of the bodice. They are more than the transition between bodice and skirt since they define the waist and often dictate how your hips will be perceived by others. There are two ways to look at waistlines—from the perspective of height, or of emphasis (since the waistline's primary effect is to emphasize or de-emphasize your hips).

Empire Waist

Raised Waist

Natural Waist

Dropped Waist

Locations

The following describes the four waistline locations and their effect on body shapes:

Empire Waist

The waist of the dress is just below the bosom (usually along the lower bra line). Emphasizes the bustline over the hips, a good choice for pear body shapes.

Raised Waist

The waist of the dress is above the body waist. Most raised waists are only 2" to 3" above the body waist. Emphasizes the midsection over the hips, a good choice for pear body shapes.

Natural Waist

The waist of the dress is in the same location as the body waist. Takes advantage of your own waistline. A good choice for hourglass body shapes.

Dropped Waist

The waist of the dress is below the body waist. Most dropped waists are only two to three inches below the body waist, although a dropped waist can occur at the hipline. A bodice with a dropped waist elongates and flatters fuller figures. It

WAISTLINE STYLES VS. BODY SHAPES

	Inverted Triangle	Hourglass	Rectangle	Pear	Round	Diamond
Asymmetrical	*	●		●	●	●
Basque		●	●		●	●
Inverted-V	●	●		●		●
Plain		●				
Straight	●	●				

* *Inverted triangle can wear a basque when combined with a strapless gown.*

CHAMEIN CANTON

emphasizes the hips over the midsection: a good choice for inverted triangle, round, and diamond body shapes. It also adds height.

Types

The type of waistline you choose will affect how the eye is drawn across your gown. We already know that it is natural human behavior to see a person from the head down. Necklines and waistlines control how fast the eye moves down the body: the square neckline slows the eye, the scoop neckline speeds the eye, and the V-neck neckline accelerates it even more. The same is true of waistlines. Waistlines that bow up—such as the inverted basque—will slow the eye, while the V-shape of the basque will speed it along. Which waistline to use depends on how much time you want the eye to linger on the waist (a very normal place for the eye to linger).

Asymmetrical

The design of the left side of the waist is not a mirror of the right side of the waist. This has a tendency to draw the eye to one side of the gown or another, forcing it to continue along an edge of the gown rather than down the center. The eye is sped along by a pronounced design. Moreover, an asymmetrical waist makes the waistline appear smaller and de-emphasizes the midsection.

Basque

The line of the waist dips in the center to form a "V." An alternative is the curved basque waistline, which dips to a "U" shape. The antebellum waist is a dropped form of the basque waist, though it is most often created using the curved basque. This waistline speeds the eye over the waist and hips. (The curved basque waist has less effect than the traditional basque waist.)

Inverted-V

An upside-down basque waist, rising in the center to form a peak. This waist style slows the eye and causes it to linger on the waist.

Plain

This gown's seamless waist is created by the cut of the cloth and no additional decoration. The line from bodice to skirt is smooth and unbroken. This style has no effect on the flow of the eye because there is no break in the gown, making it a good choice for round and diamond body shapes.

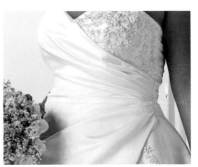
Asymmetrical Waist

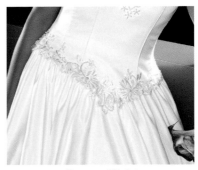
Basque Waist

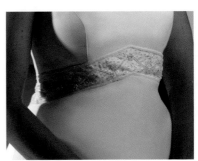
Inverted V Waist

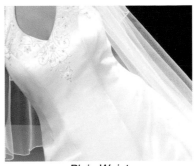
Plain Waist

Straight

A simple band around the body. This style causes the eye to pause momentarily, emphasizing the body at the location of this waist type. Pear body shapes benefit from raised and empire straight waistlines. Rectangular body shapes benefit from natural and dropped straight waistlines.

Shirred

Shirring is a feature created by folding or gathering layers of fabric into a horizontal or asymmetrical panel. While it is often referred to as a waistline, it is more accurately a decoration that can be applied at the waistline or higher, as part of the bodice. Shirring causes the eye to pause and linger, making the area where it is applied more prominent. It can even make the area appear larger.

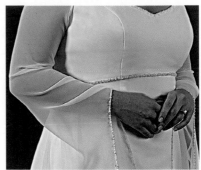
Straight Waist

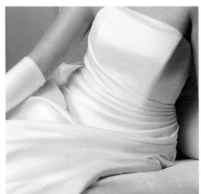
Shirred Waist

ARMS, WRISTS, AND HANDS

If I had to rate the top five areas of the body that women tend to concern themselves with the most, arms would easily be one of the highest on the list. Most of us have a love/hate relationship with our arms, which intensifies under the glare of shopping for a wedding gown. Therefore, we tend to look for gowns with sleeves that hide, distract the eye away from, or create an illusion for the arm.

Four body shapes work well with most types of sleeves: diamond, hourglass, pear, and rectangle. All four body shapes feature either a proportioned or smaller upper body (breasts, back, and upper arms) that will benefit from drawing attention towards the upper body (face, neck, and collarbone), thereby giving you more options to play with.

This isn't to say that women with round or inverted triangle body shapes can't have sleeves, but the options are fewer due to the need to pull attention away from the arms and shoulders. Remember, people see clothing (and the edges of clothing) before they see the person wearing the clothing.

Brides need to be concerned with two sleeve issues: length and type. The length of a sleeve has a dramatic effect on the apparent height and width of a woman. The type of sleeve chosen can emphasize or de-emphasize specific aspects of her body—especially the shoulders—by drawing the eye.

Sleeves vs. Straps

Do not confuse sleeves with straps. Sleeves are on your arms and can cover from your wrist up to the bend of your shoulder. Straps start at the bend of your shoulder and can cover to your neck. The primary purpose of a strap is to hold your dress up. The primary purpose of a sleeve is decoration and visual perception.

Sleeve Length

The length of the sleeve creates most of its visual bulk. The eye will be drawn to the border of the sleeve and then to the body. Thus, a full sleeve will make a woman seem taller and wider, while a short sleeve (or no sleeve) will make a woman seem shorter and thinner.

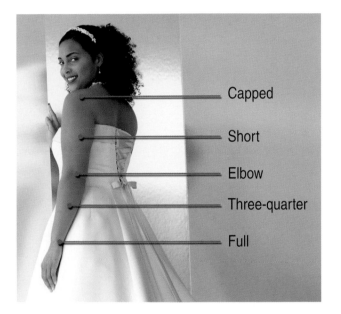

- Capped
- Short
- Elbow
- Three-quarter
- Full

SLEEVE LENGTH VS. BODY SHAPES

	Inverted Triangle	Hourglass	Rectangle	Pear	Round	Diamond
Sleeveless	?	•	•	•	•*	•
Capped		•	•	•	?	•
Short		•	•	•	?*	•
Elbow	*	•	•	•	?*	
Three Quarters	?	•	•	•	?	•
Full	•†		•		?†	•

* Make sure the sleeves are a good fit.

† Works well with illusion, but pay close attention to the sleeve's fit.

Sleeve Types

As you will see from the following illustrations, most sleeve types are designed to add bulk to the shoulders or width to a slender woman. Most full-figured women should carefully consider types other than dropped and tapered sleeves.

Bishop Sleeve

This is a very loose, flowing full sleeve gathered in at the elbow or wrist. The pear, rectangle, diamond and hourglass shapes can wear this sleeve. Keep in mind that broad shoulders will look boxy.

Cape Sleeve

This sleeve fits smoothly over the armhole and flares out at the elbow, giving the appearance of a cape. It generally looks good on hourglass, diamond, pear, and rectangle body

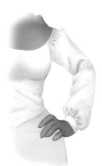

Bishop Sleeve

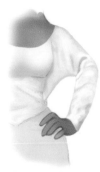

Dolman Sleeve

shapes, but does not work well on round or inverted triangle shapes. A gathered form of the cape sleeve is known as a bell sleeve.

Dolman Sleeve

This is a loose sleeve of any length. It is normally cut as an extension of the bodice and designed without a socket for the shoulder. It creates a deep, wide armhole that starts at or slightly above the waist and narrows to a point on the arm or wrist, depending on length. Loose sleeves work for most body shapes. The fit is important in determining the overall look.

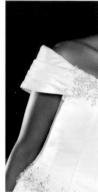

Dropped Sleeve

Dropped Sleeve

This is any sleeve (length or type) that does not enclose the shoulder. It is good for smaller upper body shapes, although it may draw attention to larger or thicker biceps. (The contessa sleeve is a dropped, short, often puffed sleeve.)

Fitted Sleeve

Any sleeve length that is cut to fit from shoulder to cuff. A sleeve that is fitted from elbow to wrist is said to be *tapered*. This sleeve draws attention to the arms. Good for slimmer upper body shapes like rectangle, diamond, pear, and hourglass.

Gigot Sleeve

This style is also known as the leg-of-mutton sleeve. It is very loose and formed like a pouf from shoulder to elbow and then tapered to the wrist. The gigot has the longest pouf of the three puffed sleeves (gigot, melon, Juliet). It's good for thinner upper body shapes, but tends to draw attention to upper arms.

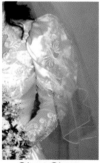

Gigot Sleeve

Juliet Sleeve

A full sleeve that is very loose and pouf-shaped from the shoulder to the upper arm and then tapered to the wrist. The Juliet sleeve (named after the costumes worn by Shakespeare's Juliet) has the shortest pouf of the three puffed sleeves (gigot, melon, Juliet). Good for thinner upper body shapes like rectangle, diamond, hourglass, and pear. On inverted triangle and round body shapes, this sleeve will draw attention to broad shoulders and the upper arms.

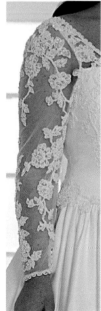

Fitted Sleeve

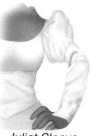

Juliet Sleeve

Melon Sleeve

A very loose and pouf-shaped sleeve from the shoulder to the middle of the upper arm, leaving the forearm bare. The size of this sleeve's pouf is midway between the Juliet and the gigot. It is good for thinner upper body shapes like rectangle, diamond, hourglass, and pear. It will draw attention to broad shoulders and upper arms on inverted triangle and round body shapes.

Poet Sleeve

A poet sleeve is fitted at the top and flares evenly from the elbow to the wrist. It can be gathered into a cuff. This sleeve works well for women with narrow hips.

Renaissance Sleeve

A long sleeve usually loosely fitted from the shoulder to the elbow that widens dramatically from the elbow, leaving the wrist free. The *butterfly* sleeve is a modified renaissance sleeve that has been split along the arm from the elbow to the cuff, giving the impression of butterfly wings. Good for thinner upper body shapes like rectangle, diamond, hourglass, and pear. On inverted triangle and round shapes, this style will draw attention to broad shoulders and the upper arms.

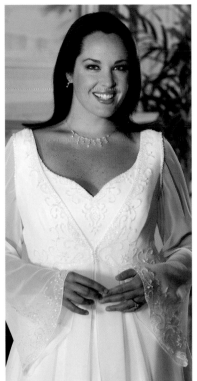

Poet Sleeve

Straight Sleeve

This is the sleeve usually found on women's and men's shirts. This is not a sleeve commonly used with wedding gowns.

Tapered Sleeve

A full sleeve that is loose from shoulder to elbow, then tapers to the wrist. Good for thinner upper bodies. Round and inverted triangle body shapes may be able to wear this sleeve because it is loose from the shoulders.

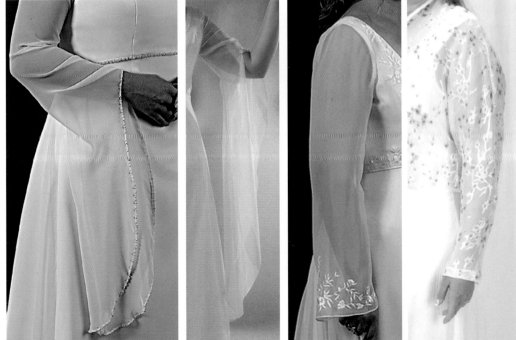

Renaissance, Butterfly, Straight, and Tapered Sleeves

Tulip Sleeve

A cap or short sleeve made of overlapping folds of cloth to form a tulip shape. Overlapping folds look attractive on thinner upper body shapes. On round and inverted triangle body shapes, however, it adds width and draws negative attention to the arms.

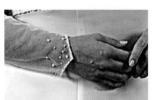

Tulip Sleeve

Illusion and Sleeves

Illusion netting is often used to modify the visible effect sleeves have on the body. It allows women whose body shapes generally don't lend themselves well to sleeves the ability to have sleeves. It also softens the visibility of sleeves on women who need them, but would rather emphasize another part of their body. Shorter sleeve lengths can be worn by hourglass, rectangle, pear, and diamond shapes. Longer illusion sleeves work well with round and inverted triangle shapes since they serve to elongate the arms while de-emphasizing broad shoulders or large upper arm areas.

Cuffs

Cuffs are the hemline of the sleeve. They are used both to decorate and to draw the eye toward or away from your wrists and hands. Generally, the more decorative the cuff, the more attention it draws.

Fitted Cuff

The cuff is cut to fit snugly around the wrist or arm. It is best used to draw attention to slender wrists or toned arms.

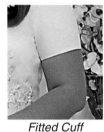

Fitted Cuff

Poet Cuff

The cuff flares at the wrist, usually uniformly, to cover the back of the hand. The butterfly cuff is a modification of the poet cuff in which the cuff is split from wrist to hem and often elongated along the bottom to create the effect of butterfly wings. The poet and butterfly cuffs look good on most body shapes. They tend to make the hands appear longer, and are styles often associated with romance.

Pointed Cuff

Pointed Cuff

This is a fitted cuff that has been drawn to a V-shaped point over the back of the hand. It is a good choice if you have shapely hands.

Scalloped Cuff

A fitted or straight cuff that has a scalloped edge. It is most commonly used with shorter sleeves and draws attention to the arms.

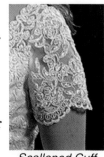

Scalloped Cuff

Straight Cuff

A common cuff, loose on the arm or wrist with a straight edge. Draws the least attention to the arm or wrist.

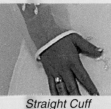
Straight Cuff

Gloves

Not all brides choose to wear gloves, but for those who do, the following information will act as a guideline.

Gloves come in varying lengths and are generally worn with gowns having elbow-length sleeves or shorter. Gloves should be avoided with long-sleeve gowns.

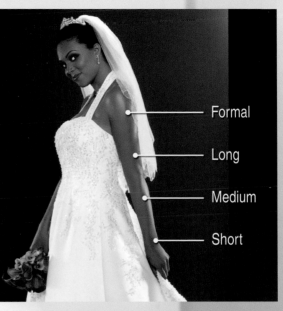

- *Short:* zero to one button glove. Wrist length gloves work best with short-sleeved gowns.

- *Medium* (ranging between the wrist and the elbow): two and four button gloves. Frequently used with cap sleeve gowns.

- *Long:* over-the-elbow gloves. Should be worn with sleeveless or strapless gowns.

- *Formal:* opera gloves that go further up the arms to the area of the biceps. Should be worn with sleeveless or strapless gowns.

Many short gloves are of lace or illusion. Longer gloves are often silk or satin. For crepe gowns, choose a cotton glove.

Short gloves are good for both informal and semiformal events. They draw the eye away from the shoulders and bustline and focus it on the wrist and forearm. Fingerless gloves take this a step further and draw the eye to your fingers.

Over-the-elbow gloves aren't a good choice for brides with large upper arms since they emphasize that particular area. They are a good choice for women with a pear shaped body because they will widen the appearance of the upper body. Wearing over-the-elbow gloves will shorten the appearance of the arms on petite women.

Formal gloves (often called opera gloves) work best for women with toned arms due to their length and their need to fit snugly to keep the glove from falling to the wrist. The overall effect of a formal glove on body height and width is similar to the effect of a long sleeve. They will make the upper body appear wider while de-emphasizing the upper arms. However, where the cuff of a long sleeve will cause the eye to pause near the hips, formal gloves will cause the eye to pause near the bosom. For this reason, a shapely bosom is recommended with formal gloves.

A note about hands. If you are blessed with pianist hands (long fingers, great dexterity) then most gloves will look great. Just make sure you balance them with your upper arms. (For additional information on gloves, see the Glossary.)

VEILS

One of the most hallowed components of a wedding ensemble is the veil. Let's face it, one of the highlights of the wedding ceremony occurs when the groom lifts the veil and kisses the bride. What could be more beautiful?

The fact is, while it may seem that choosing a wedding veil should be a simple task, in reality it isn't. Just like your wedding gown, there are many factors involved when deciding which type of veil will work best for you. Three specific issues to consider are face shape, body shape, and your back. We need to compare these to the three basic aspects of veil design: shape, length, and type.

General Advice

Before committing yourself to any particular type or length of veil, visit a bridal salon and try some veils on using their three-sided mirrors. The mirrors will give you an idea of how the veil looks from many angles, including some rear views. Wear a dress when you do this because slacks or jeans will throw off the view of your hips and thighs. If you think one of the longer, heavier veils is right for you, ask the salon to let you try on a dress appropriate for the veil (any dress, you don't need to look your best in it) and walk the store's length a few times. Make sure the weight of the veil pulling against your neck is comfortable—remember how long your wedding day will be.

After this, if you're still committed to a long veil, make sure you think through your entire wedding day. Be sure your *day* can handle your veil. Will you be in a stretch limo or a sedan? Will you be outside in the wind or inside in a small room? Your veil needs to compliment your beauty, but it also needs to fit within the world of your wedding day.

Face Shapes

The first aspect we will consider is the shape of your face. Face shapes generally fall into two categories: curved shapes (oval, round, oblong, heart/inverted triangle), and angular shapes (square, rectangle, diamond, triangle/pear).

Face shapes are basically defined using the width of the face measured cheekbone to cheekbone, the length of the face measured from hairline to chin, the height of the cheekbone line, and the strength of the jawline. Curved shapes generally have slender jawlines while angular shapes generally have strong jawlines. To determine the shape of your face, pull your hair away from your face and pay close attention to the outline and details of the edges.

Now we'll look at face shapes individually:

Oval Face

The face is longer than it is wide, with the cheekbone height obviously above the midpoint of the face and a slender jawline. This is an all-purpose shape that can be complimented by most veils.

Round Face

Face length and width are approximately equal; cheekbone height is close to the midpoint of the face with a slender jawline. The face wants to be framed, but avoid layers (cascade veils), which will widen the face.

Oblong Face

The face is longer than it is wide, but the cheekbone height is close to the midpoint of the face with a slender jawline. This shape wants bulk around the mid-face to make it appear wider. Cascade veils work best. Avoid a straight veil, as that will make the face look longer.

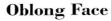

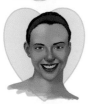

Heart/Inverted Triangle Face

This shape usually has wide eyes or an unusually slender jawline. The forehead is wide. Use veil bulk to add width to the bottom of the face, but avoid adding width to the mid-face. A back veil will work best to achieve this.

Square Face

Face length and width are approximately equal. Cheekbone height is close to the midpoint of the face and the face has a strong jawline. Use long, narrow veils to draw attention away from the face. Avoid short, bulky veils that make the face more pronounced.

Rectangular Face

Face is longer than it is wide with a strong jawline. A long veil will soften the jaw, whereas shorter veils make the jawline appear more pronounced.

Diamond Face

Face length and width are approximately equal; cheekbone height is close to the midpoint of the face with a slender jawline. A diamond effect is created either by pronounced cheekbones or by the combination of a narrow forehead and slender jawline. This is an all-purpose shape that can be complimented by most veils.

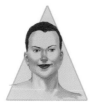

Pear/Triangle Face

This facial shape is characterized by a narrow forehead, wide jawline, and a wide chin. The object here is to build fullness through the narrow portion of the face. Use veil bulk to add width to the forehead and through the eyes, but avoid adding width to the jawline.

Veil Shapes

The basics of veil design are best understood if you start by laying the cloth out flat on a floor. The shape of the cloth will determine how the edge of the cloth hangs down your back. The pick point (the point in the cloth where you attach the veil to the head piece) will determine bulk, line, and flare. You can pick the center of the cloth, an edge, a corner, or anywhere in between. Picking a point somewhere off the fabric edge creates a cascade veil. The pick point's distance from the fabric edge will determine the widest point of the veil.

The following veil shapes are defined independently from their lengths. Thus, a veil is said to be a square-cut veil even if its length makes it resemble a rectangle.

Oval Veil

The veil is cut in a circle or oval creating a distinctive cloth gather at the bottom of the veil. This veil flares around the face and tends to fall uniformly down the back and has the least bulk at its widest point. This is a good choice for oval, oblong, heart, and triangular face shapes.

Diamond Veil

The veil is cut in a square or rectangle with a pick-point along the fabric's diagonal axis. This veil widens (bulks) dramatically early in its fall, then tapers sharply to its end point. It has the greatest bulk at its widest point of the three veil shapes. A good choice for rectangle, square, and diamond face shapes.

Square Veil

The veil is cut in a square or rectangle with a pick-point along the fabric's square axis. This veil's widest point is always at or near the bottom of the veil. It's flare is strong, but slender. A good choice for oblong and triangular face shapes.

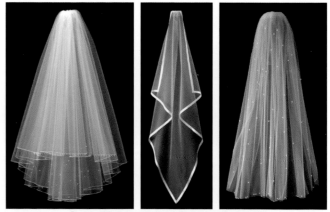

Oval, Diamond, and Square Cut Veils

Lengths

In general, veil lengths affect how tall you look. However, veils at the extremes (very short and very long) have extra considerations. Most of a veil's bulk is at the lower end of the veil, so a short veil will bring that bulk above your waist or even to your shoulders. Wide faces should avoid short veils. On the other hand, the bulk of a long veil is on the floor, dragging behind you. This exposes your back to the world. Full-figured brides should also keep in mind that a long, clean cut veil will elongate the entire look of their wedding ensemble.

A quick note about stock vs. custom veils. A custom veil will be cut to meet your exact body measurements. A stock veil will be cut to a length

VEIL LENGTH VS. BODY SHAPES

	Inverted Triangle	Hourglass	Rectangle	Pear	Round	Diamond
Shoulder		•		•		•
Elbow		•	•	•		
Waist	•	•	•			
Fingertip	•	•				
Knee	•	•	•			•
Ballet (Waltz)	•	•	•	•	•	•
Sweep	•	•	•	•	•	•
Chapel	•	•				•
Cathedral	•	•	•		•	•
Royal Cathedral	•	•	•			

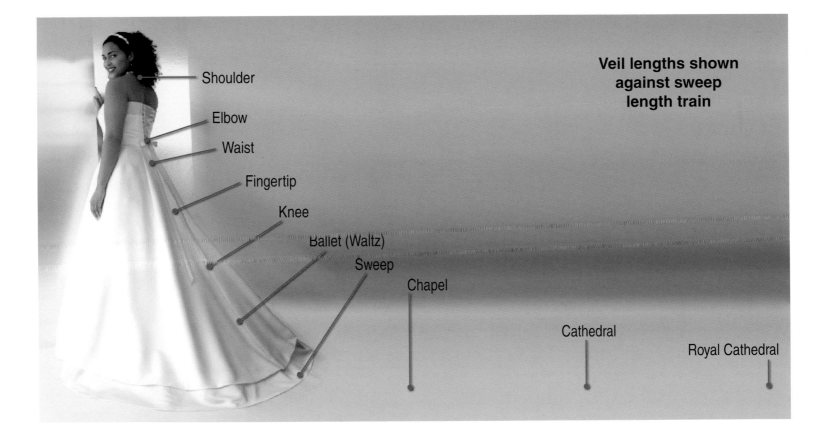

Shoulder
Elbow
Waist
Fingertip
Knee
Ballet (Waltz)
Sweep
Chapel
Cathedral
Royal Cathedral

Veil lengths shown against sweep length train

in inches that approximates the standard body measurements, but may differ by several inches from custom lengths.

Shoulder Length Veil

The lower end of the veil falls just above the shoulders (stock length: 18"–24"). This veil flares dramatically around the neck and shoulders and makes the face more pronounced. It focuses attention on the upper body, making you appear taller, but also broadening the shoulders.

Elbow/Waist Length Veil

The lower end of the veil falls to the elbows or waist of your dress (stock length: 24"–38"). This veil is essentially neutral, but for round and diamond body shapes, it will draw attention to the midsection.

Fingertip Length Veil

The lower end of the veil falls to the tips of your index fingers when you are standing straight with your arms to your sides and your hands outstretched (stock length: 38"–40"). This veil focuses attention on your midsection, making it appear wider.

Knee Length Veil

The lower end of the veil falls to your knees (stock length: 40"–50"). This veil focuses attention on your hips, making them appear wider. This veil gives your body an overall appearance of being shorter. It is not a good choice for pear shapes or round shapes with shorter legs.

Ballet (Waltz) Length Veil

The lower end of the veil falls to the calves, or the midpoint between the knees and the ankles (stock length: 50"–60"). This veil focuses attention on your lower legs: a good choice for round and pear body shapes that want a longer veil (although in this case they should avoid a diamond cut veil).

Sweep Length Veil

The lower end of the veil falls to the floor (stock length: 60"–72"). This veil frames the entire body. It is best suited for hourglass and rectangle body shapes. It gives the body an overall appearance of being shorter.

Chapel Length Veil

The lower end of the veil extends behind the gown by two to three feet when the bride is standing still (stock length: 72"–90"). This veil will pull away from your back when you walk, but usually settles on the back when you stop (depending on floor friction). The effect is to encompass the back, emphasizing the hips. Not a good choice for round, pear, or diamond body shapes.

Cathedral Length Veil

The lower end of the veil extends behind the gown by three to five feet when the bride is standing still (stock length: 108"–140"). This veil is often connected at the shoulders or waist and combined with another veil due to its weight. It will pull away from your back when you walk and stay that way when you stop unless helped. It usually requires attendants to monitor where the veil is when you walk. This is a beautiful veil, but if you're planning on an outdoor wedding or ceremony, be careful of Mother Nature (wind, etc.). Good for all shapes except the pear, which will suffer for the extra visual bulk extending from the hips.

> When the cathedral or royal cathedral length veils are used without a train, they are often described as a watteau or capelet train.

Royal Cathedral Length Veil

Also known as either a regal or a monarch veil. The lower end of the veil extends behind the gown by five to eight feet when the bride is standing still (stock length: 140"–180"). This veil is often connected at the shoulders or waist and combined with another veil due to its weight. Most wedding locations are not built to handle veils of this length, so brides should avoid this veil unless they have a very long walk to the altar. This veil will pull away from your back when you walk and stay that way without help when you stop. It usually requires attendants to monitor where the veil is when you walk. This is a gorgeous veil, but weighs quite a lot. If you truly want this veil, be sure your headpiece isn't too heavy—and again, be careful of Mother Nature.

Types

To paraphrase the Bard, a veil by any other name is still a veil. This is true, but the type of veil you choose will have an impact on how you are perceived by people. The following illustrations depict the effects the different veil types create, and indicate which face and body types work best with a given style:

Angel Veil

A square cut veil that flares out from the headpiece and over the shoulders with the appearance of angel's wings. A good choice for short veils (fingertip and shorter), but the effect is generally lost with longer veils due to their weight. Dramatically widens the face and emphasizes the shoulders. Good for oblong faces and pear body shapes.

Back Veil

The veil is connected to a narrow point at the back of the head, creating a very narrow look from the head to below the shoulders. Has no effect on body shape when viewed from the front. Can make a broad back appear narrower by drawing attention to the center of the back. A good choice for heart- and diamond-shaped faces and inverted triangle body shapes.

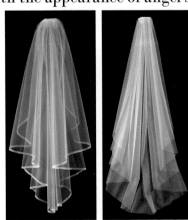

Angel and Back Veils

Birdcage Veil

This is not a traditional veil. It is a hat or comb with a blusher that is usually not designed to be thrown back over the head, but rather lifted for the kiss. Widens the forehead and draws attention away from the shoulders and back. A good choice for diamond-shaped faces and round body shapes.

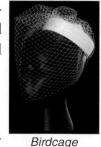

Birdcage

Butterfly Veil

An oval cut veil that flares out from the headpiece and over the shoulders with the appearance of butterfly wings. A good choice for short veils (waist and shorter), but the effect is generally lost with longer veils due to their weight. Dramatically widens the face and emphasizes the shoulders. Good for oblong faces and pear body shapes.

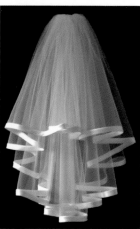

Butterfly

Flyaway Veil

A shoulder length cascade veil made of stiff illusion that flares dramatically to the sides and back of the bride. Dramatically widens the face. Should only be used with oblong faces, especially with pear or round body shapes.

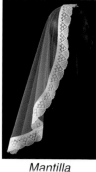

Flyaway

Fountain Veil

The most common type of veil. Moderately widens the face, but usually falls within the shoulder width, so there is no impact on the shoulders. The primary consideration is the veil length and the associated apparent height change.

Fountain

Mantilla Veil

A square or oval cut veil that is draped over the head. Dramatically widens and lengthens the face; tends to widen shoulders and shorten the neck. Best used by brides with square faces, long necks, and a pear body shape.

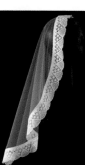

Mantilla

Back Drape

Perhaps not thought of traditionally as a veil, a back drape is a solid fabric (not veil illusion) that drapes from the shoulders or the waist to the floor. It often takes the place of a veil and is reminiscent of the long, heavy robes worn by medieval monarchy. Today, they are often satin-backed velvet. A back drape that extends beyond the hem of the gown is known as a Watteau train.

Attributes

Veil attributes are features that can be added to any veil type.

Pouf

A pouf or veil pouf is a popular head decoration, although it is not considered a headpiece. Veil illusion is gathered to create a pouf and sits atop the veil and headpiece. It has the effect of making the body seem taller and the face longer.

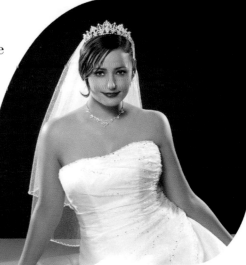

Ornamentation

Pearls, brilliants, and various edgings, can be added to enhance and individualize any veil. (See Veil Design in the Glossary for edging suggestions.)

Pouf

Blusher

A blusher is a piece of veil illusion that is pulled over a portion or over all of the bride's face. On a traditional veil, the blusher becomes the top tier of a cascade. A non-traditional blusher would be a non-removable piece of illusion attached to the forward brim of a hat.

Cascade (Tiered)

A cascade veil is created when two or more layers of illusion fall in a tiered or layered fashion. Fountain veils with a pick-point away from the fabric edge are naturally cascaded veils. Cascades can also be created by adding layers of illusion fabric. Face shapes that need extra bulk to widen the apparent width of the face should use cascade veils. Face shapes that do not want the extra bulk should avoid them.

Headpieces

Headpieces draw attention up the face to the forehead, and have the ability to widen the forehead or lengthen the face. They are also the means of attaching all but the longest veils, which means they must bear weight. As the veil becomes larger (either by design or length), the headpiece must become larger and sturdier, which will impact the shape of the face.

Note that most headpieces can be worn with or without a veil.

Backpiece

Sometimes called a back spray, a backpiece is any headpiece worn on the back of the head. It is used to attach a veil that does not frame the face. Backpieces are one of the weakest headpieces and should not be used to attach a heavily cascaded veil or a veil longer than fingertip length. Backpieces remove the effect veils have on the sides of the head and let the veil frame the neck. For heart-shaped and triangle-shaped faces, it takes attention away from the widest point of the face. For diamond and rectangle body shapes, it draws attention away from the midsection when the bride is viewed from the side.

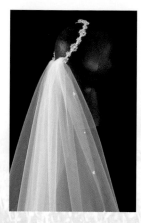

Bun Ring

A subtype of crown, a bun ring is worn around hair pulled into a bun rather than around the crown of the head. Bun rings can be thin, surrounding the base of the bun, or wide to encapsulate the bun. They draw attention to the top of the head. The degree depends on where the hair bun is created. Wider bun rings draw the eye more strongly. They will lengthen the body and the face. Bun rings are only as strong as your hair bun. Worn high on the head, they have great strength; worn low at the back, they can slip off if not secured well. Most face shapes can wear some form of a bun. Talk to your hairdresser to see what will work best for you.

Cap

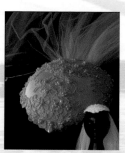

This headpiece is larger than a headband, but smaller than a hat. A cap is usually a decorated cover for the crown of the head. (A specific type of cap is the Juliet cap.) It is used to attach veils of moderate length (up to sweep length—possibly chapel length). Because they fit close to the head they do not lengthen the body, but they will widen the forehead. Not a good choice for round, heart-shaped, or square-shaped faces.

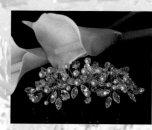

Comb

A hair comb used to attach the veil or a spray. When worn on the back of the head, it is called a backpiece. This is a common means of attaching a veil. Combs have little effect on face and body shape. However, they are generally weak and should not be used to attach a veil longer than fingertip length. Combs can be worn by all face shapes.

Crown

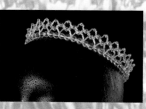

A circular headpiece worn on the crown of the head. Crowns have a uniform height around their circumference. They draw the eye to the top of the head, lengthening the face and making the body appear taller. Choose a crown that fits your head and face without adding bulk.

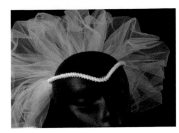

Halo

A band worn over the forehead that ties or connects at the back of the head. Wreaths and V-bands are specific types of halos. This headpiece draws attention to the forehead without weighting it, and will make the face look somewhat smaller without widening the forehead. Halos have good strength and can hold all but the longest veils.

Hat

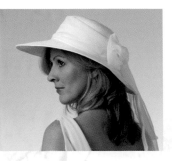

The largest of the headpieces, hats differ from caps primarily because they have a brim. Hats have the most significant effect on face and body shape because they are visually heavy. This makes them good for pear-shaped bodies, but a poor choice for heart- or square-shaped faces. Hats can bear the most weight of any headpiece, though the longer veil lengths should still be avoided.

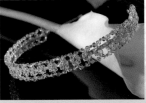

Headband

A thin band worn over the crown of the head and over or behind the ears. Veils attached along the band's length have a mantilla look without weighing heavily over the shoulders. The headband itself has no impact on face or body shape, but it will cause the veil to spread out across the back, framing the lower face.

Spray

Sometimes called a side spray, it is any decorative piece worn on the side of the head. Sprays cause the forehead to appear wider, but the asymmetry of the spray makes it a good choice for oblong faces as it draws the eye to a side of the head. The line of sight must then cross the mid-face to continue down the dress. Veils do not connect to sprays. Not good for round, heart-shaped, or triangle-shaped faces.

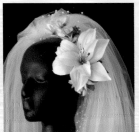

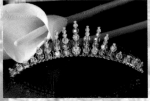

Tiara

A circular headpiece worn on the crown of the head. The height of a tiara rises to a peak at the front. It is visibly less weighty than a crown. This headpiece is a good choice for brides who want a top-of-head headpiece without the drawbacks of the crown or bun ring. Like the hat and crown, tiaras can carry good veil weight. They are generally a good choice for all face shapes.

SKIRTS

The basic shape of your skirt was determined when you selected your silhouette, but we still need to discuss skirt length (hemline) and type (accessories), and your train. Your choice of skirt and train will affect your apparent height, and will also affect the way you are seen from the back and the side.

Hemlines

Wedding skirts have been made in all hem lengths. However, the higher the hem, the less common it is for a gown. Street and intermission lengths are more common for bridesmaids and second marriages. Minis are more common for rock stars and celebrity weddings—definitely not for the faint of heart.

Brides should think long and hard before deciding on a hemline other than floor or ballet—and they should review their decision if they choose ballet—because any hem other than the floor hem will draw the eye away from the upper body. Remember that the eye is drawn to edges of things, so a hemline off the floor will cause the eye to slide off your skirt and stop to linger on whatever is right below the hem.

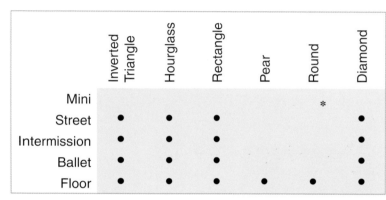

	Inverted Triangle	Hourglass	Rectangle	Pear	Round	Diamond
Mini					*	
Street	●	●	●			●
Intermission	●	●	●			●
Ballet	●	●	●			●
Floor	●	●	●	●	●	●

* *Round body shapes blessed with shapely legs can benefit from a street-length hemline because it will draw the eye quickly from the body's midsection.*

Remember, you'll be on your feet for eight to twelve hours. Most people don't spend more than two hours on their feet in a day, and that's spread over the entire day. Your feet, ankles, and lower legs will swell by the end of your wedding day, and that much accumulated water and blood can cause edema and other skin discolorations. Before you set your heart on a hem other than a floor hem, spend an entire day on your feet in shoes similar to those you will be wearing on your wedding day, and then examine your legs to be sure they'll pass the public exam.

One final consideration: keep in mind that the higher the hemline, the more limited your options will be for including a train with your gown.

Mini Hemline

Measured from the waist to a point above the knees. Will make the body appear taller by focusing attention on the hips and legs, and should not be worn by anyone that doesn't have perfect hips and legs.

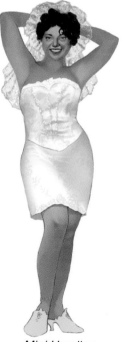

Mini Hemline

CHAMEIN CANTON

Street Hemline

Also known as knee length. Measured from the waist to a point at or just below the knees. Will make the body appear taller by focusing attention on the knees. Good for rectangle, hourglass, and diamond body shapes, or round shapes if the bride has shapely legs.

Intermission Hemline

Also known as tea and midi length. Measured to a point midway between the knees and ankles. Will make the body appear somewhat taller by focusing attention on the calf and ankles. Good for diamond, hourglass, and rectangle shapes since they tend to be leggier.

Ballet Hemline

Also known as ballerina length. Measured from the waist to the ankles. Generally neutral. Focuses attention on the ankles and feet.

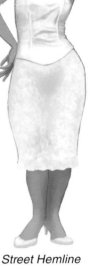

Street Hemline

Floor Hemline

The most common hemline. Measured from the waist to the floor (or a fraction of an inch above it). Will make the body appear shorter, but allows the eye to sweep from your waist down without stopping. The result is that most people will focus on your upper body.

Hi-Lo Hemline

The hi-lo hemline is created when one portion of the hemline is higher than the rest of the hem. Hi-lo hems are usually high in the front or on one side.

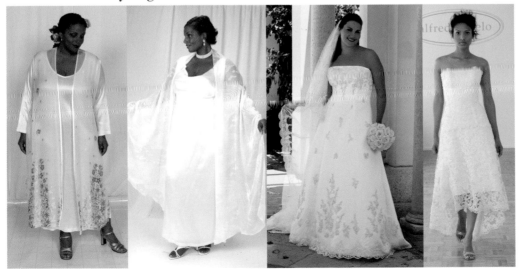

In general, the longer and shapelier your legs, the higher your hemline can be. The Skirt Attributes vs. Body Shapes table tells you which hemlines generally work well with which body shapes, but the table presumes you have the longer, shapelier legs to go with the higher hemlines. When in doubt, go with a lower hemline.

Intermission, Ballet, Floor, and Hi-Lo Hemlines

SKIRTS

Skirt Attributes

Skirt attributes describe the various accessories and decorations used on a skirt. Skirt attributes primarily affect how you are seen from the sides and back. Your goal with the skirt attributes is to choose attributes that balance you in these directions.

Apron

An overskirt that closes at the back of the waist. Draws attention to the front of the body, reducing the visible impact of the buttocks. Not good for body shapes seeking to take attention away from the lower body.

Bouffant (Bouffant Draped Skirt)

A sheer, puffed-out skirt often made of stiffened silk, rayon, or nylon net. It blurs the edge of the skirt, but also adds bulk to the skirt. It is often very full with a hoop slip, and is generally only used by the ball silhouette. The bouffant can also be draped to the side of the skirt creating an asymmetrical waistline. (This can also be referred to as a cascading skirt.) This is a good way for inverted triangles and rectangles to build up their hips in order to balance the upper and lower body.

SKIRT ATTRIBUTES VS. BODY SHAPES

	Inverted Triangle	Hourglass	Rectangle	Pear	Round	Diamond
Apron	•	•	•	*		•
Bouffant	•	•	•	?		•
Bow	•	•	•			
Box Pleated		•		• *		•
Bustle	•	•		?		•
Flounce	•	•			•	•
Fluted		•	•			•
Pannier	•	•	•			
Peplum	•	•	•			
Pick Up	•	•	•			•
Redingote	•	•		•		•
Tiered	•	•	•		•	•
Trumpet		•				•

* Use of this skirt effect depends on the amount and type of material. For pear shapes, too much material will add bulk to the lower body.

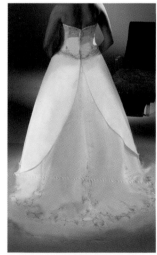

Apron

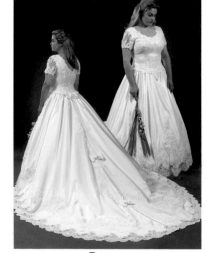

Bouffant Skirt

Bows

Bow

A large bow placed at the back of the waist. Draws attention to the back of the gown and the backside. Not good for those seeking to slim an ample backside.

Box Pleated Skirt

A skirt with deep pleats of parallel fabric folds. The pleats usually start at the natural waist. Tends to make the hips and legs appear more slender. Should be avoided if your midsection, hips or buttocks will pull at the pleats. The effect is stronger than for the fluted skirt.

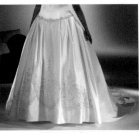
Box Pleated Skirt

Bustle

A gather of cloth at the back of the waist. It is often created by gathering a length of train and attaching it at the waist. Adds to the backside. Elongates the buttocks both front-to-back and top-to-bottom. Has a stronger effect than a peplum or a redingote. Most bustles are detachable. (See Glossary for details.)

Flounce

A wide piece of cloth (sometimes ruffled) attached to the hem of a skirt. Often used decoratively with ballet length skirts to create a floor length skirt. Gently draws the eyes down the skirt. Shortens overall height and de-emphasizes the upper body.

Fluted Skirt

A gathered skirt producing vertical grooves when hanging straight. Tends to make the hips and legs appear more slender. Should be avoided if your hips or buttocks will pull at the folds. Effect is weaker than for the box pleated skirt. Good for hourglass shapes.

Fluted Skirt

Overskirt

A layer of cloth producing the look of one skirt lying atop another. Aprons and redingotes are specific types of overskirts. (Tiered skirts are created using multiple overskirts.)

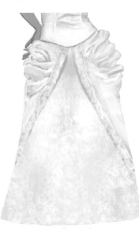
Pannier

Pannier

Gathered fabric worn on the hips over the skirt to produce a scalloped look. Widens the hips without emphasizing the buttocks. A good choice for inverted triangles.

Peplum

A short length (or lengths) of cloth attached to the back of the skirt that is often layered to create a cascade effect leading to the train. Elongates the buttocks both front-to-back in a side view, and top-to-bottom when viewed from the back. Has a weaker effect than a bustle, but a stronger effect than a redingote.

SKIRTS

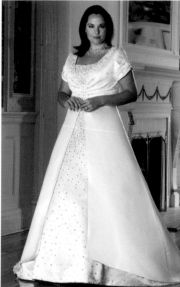
Redingote

Pickup Skirt

The fabric of the skirt is drawn up at four to six points around the circumference of the skirt at about mid-thigh to create a scalloped effect. Draws the eye below the hips and causes it to linger. A good way of de-emphasizing broad shoulders without affecting apparent height.

Redingote (Redingcote)

Visually the reverse of a smooth-fitting apron that flares and may or may not flow into a train behind the dress. It also refers to an over-skirt that fastens in front, a woman's lightweight coat that is open down the front, or a dress with a front gore of contrasting material. Elongates the buttocks both front-to-back in a side view, and top-to-bottom when viewed from the back. Has a weaker effect than a bustle or a peplum.

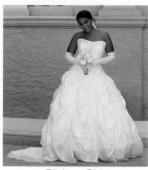
Pickup Skirt

Tiered Skirt

A skirt constructed of overlapping layers of fabric of varying lengths. Emphasizes the lower body without adding bulk. A good choice for inverted triangle and rectangle body shapes.

Trumpet Skirt

A skirt that flares from the knees to the hem in the shape of a trumpet's bell. A trumpet skirt is the centerpiece of the mermaid silhouette. Draws the eye dramatically to the lower legs with the effect of actually de-emphasizing the upper body. Requires shapely legs. Good for hourglass shapes.

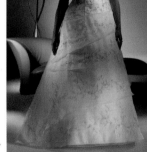
Tiered Skirt

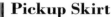

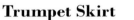
Trumpet Skirt

TRAINS

One of the most dramatic elements of a bridal gown is one of the last things people see when the bride goes by— the train. It's an essential part of every woman's fairy tale wedding event. However, when it comes to choosing a train, body shape and height make the difference in how the train will look and feel.

Generally speaking, you want to make sure your train is proportionate to your height and body shape. For example, a petite pear-shaped bride would look lovely with a chapel or even semi-cathedral train. Neither would completely overpower her. On the other hand, if she were to choose a cathedral train, it would add weight and width to the bottom of the gown. A tall pear shape, however, would have the height to carry a cathedral train.

Conversely, for tall brides with an hourglass shape, a sweep train may prove to be a bit too short —especially if they're wearing heels. In this case, a chapel train would be a good choice.

Most trains are designed to be removed after the ceremony, so if you do opt for a long train, you're not stuck dragging it around during the reception. Nevertheless, you will spend a good portion of the day with it. Think about it. Study the following illustrations and make your decision from there.

TRAINS VS. BODY SHAPE and TYPE

Table indicates whether each train is appropriate for (P) petite, (A) average, or (T) tall women given a particular body shape

	Inverted Triangle	Hourglass	Rectangle	Pear	Round	Diamond
Sweep	PA	PA	PA	PA	PA	PA
Court	PAT	PAT	PAT	PAT	PAT	PAT
Chapel	PAT	PAT	PAT	PAT	PAT	PAT
Semi-cathedral	PAT	PAT	PAT	PAT	PAT	PAT
Cathedral	T		T	T		T

I've left the royal cathedral and monarch trains out of the chart. While true that long trains will generally make you look shorter, there comes a time when other factors override how the train will affect your looks. If you have the money to buy these trains, a limo that can contain these trains, a facility where the ceremony will take place that can handle these trains, enough attendants to help you maneuver these trains, and a back that can stand up under the weight of these trains, then how they affect your apparent height isn't a primary issue. But it's still worth saying that the key word here is balance.

Common Train Lengths

The following train lengths are commonly used in modern weddings. The lengths are manageable, yet still project the beauty and tradition of the ceremony. Common train lengths are also popular because many of today's ceremonies take place in locations that cannot accommodate long, formal trains.

Sweep Train

Also known as floor, duster, and brush trains. The train's length is 8"–12" measured from the hem of the skirt.

Court Train

The train's length is 12"–36" measured from the hem of the skirt.

Chapel Train

Also known as a medium train. Its length is 36"–48" measured from the hem of the skirt. This is the most common (and perhaps the most popular) train. It compliments all body types and shapes.

Semi-cathedral Train

The train's length is 48"–72" measured from the hem of the skirt.

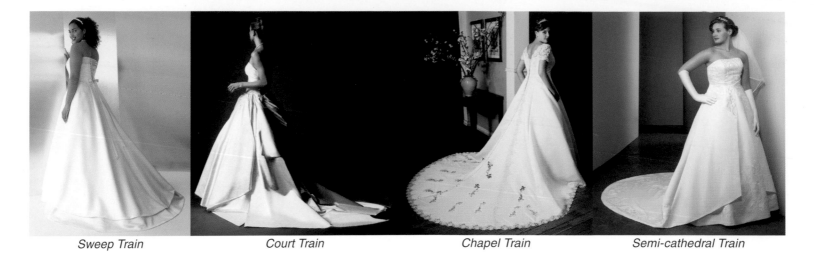

Sweep Train   Court Train   Chapel Train   Semi-cathedral Train

Formal Train Lengths

Formal train lengths are usually reserved for very formal weddings. Their cost and size contribute to their infrequent use. Brides considering formal trains must be sure that the cars they ride in, the location of their wedding, and their dressing quarters will all accommodate the bulk associated with these trains.

Brides considering formal train lengths should also be sure they are comfortable dragging the train behind them. Formal trains are usually attached at the waist rather than incorporated as part of the hem to avoid an unnatural pull on the hem when the bride walks. One of the traditional purposes of bridal attendants was to carry the train.

The infrequent use of these large trains has also contributed to the general misuse of their names.

Cathedral Train

This train's length is 72"–96" measured from the hem of the skirt.

Royal Cathedral Train

Also known as a traditional royal train. The train's length is 96"–120" measured from the hem of the skirt.

Monarch Train

Also known as a royal train (not to be confused with the royal cathedral or traditional royal train). This train is usually reserved for wealthy, formal weddings and, of course, monarchs. The train's length is 144" or more measured from the hem of the skirt.

The Watteau Train

Also known as a capelet train. This is any train that attaches at the shoulders rather than being an elongation of the hem of the skirt. The watteau train is an elegant looking train well suited for the medium train lengths. When shorter train lengths are used, it is more often called a back drape. The longer train lengths will cause the bride to stoop or lean forward as she walks. If you are considering a long watteau train you should take the time to test its weight to be sure you can walk comfortably upright.

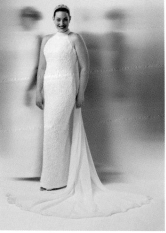
Watteau Train

BOLEROS

A loose jacket or coat that is open at the front is called a bolero. Bolero jackets can be fingertip length, waist length, or fall just below the bustline. The duster-like coat is usually three-quarter or floor length. Boleros can be constructed of any fabric, but are particularly attractive with wedding attire when made of a sheer fabric, embroidered or plain.

Short boleros can be worn with any silhouette. The longer bolero jackets and coats produce a thinning effect when layered over column, sheath, or tank style dresses. Their overall long lines and the layered look they produce tend to balance the body by de-emphasizing large busts, waists, or hips.

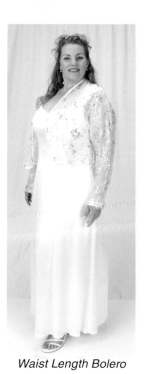
Waist Length Bolero

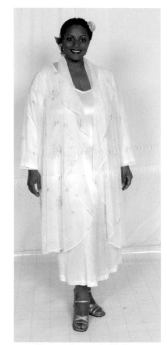
Fingertip Length Bolero

Street Length Bolero

Intermission Length Bolero

FABRIC

Fabric texture is an intrinsic part of the design for any piece of clothing, from dress to business suit. A change in fabric can, in fact, give the item a completely different look. So when it comes to your wedding gown, choosing the right fabric is essential.

Full-figured women have an extra consideration in choosing fabric. According to Peggy Lutz of Peggy Lutz Designs, "Hard fabrics look good on hard little bodies. Traditional satin is the worst choice for plus-size brides because it doesn't give."

Full-figured women need soft fabrics that will help accentuate their curves and emphasize the positive. Their choice of fabric, therefore, is just as important—if not more so—than the gown design itself.

As you begin thumbing through bridal catalogs or magazines, avoid the common mistake of glancing at the overall picture and making an impulsive decision. Instead, take time to consider the cut and detail of each gown based on what you have learned in the previous sections. Then ask yourself:

- What type of fabric was used to make the dress?

- Is it the best fabric choice for my body?

Gowns are made of everything from heavy satins to chiffon. Select fabrics that feel best on you and work well with the dress style you have chosen. In light of the number of choices available, it's a good idea to take a test drive. Visit a bridal salon and try on dresses made from different fabrics. Pay close attention to the way each fabric drapes. Is it comfortable? Does the fabric give to hug your curves like a favorite sweater, or is it stiff and unyielding? How does it make your skin look? Glowing or sallow? These aspects are important if you want to play up the curves and skin that got his attention in the first place!

If you need an objective second opinion about how a fabric looks on you, don't be afraid to ask the salon's consultant. Most consultants have seen every fabric on every shape. They will be able to advise you on what is or isn't working for you.

In the end, however, you should rely on your own two eyes. After all, it's your body, and who knows it better than you? Most of us have a good idea of what works on our body; we simply need the self-confidence to go with it! In the end, you're the one who will be wearing the gown—and you need to feel comfortable in it!

COLOR

For most brides, the choice of color for their wedding gown is simple—white. White is an elegant color. It can be worn by all skin shades, be they African American, Asian, Caucasian, Indian, or Latino. However, brides must take special care when designing gowns and accessories because white is never actually white.

The color white has many shades, and these shades are complicated by the sheen and texture of different fabrics (generally more so than any other color). Some of the shades you will encounter are:

White	*Cream*	*Linen*
Off White	*Eggshell*	*Seashell*
Antique White	*Champagne*	*Snow*
Floral White	*Old Lace*	*Ivory*

Shades of white will generally have yellow or gray undertones. Since you will look better if you have a little contrast between your skin and the fabric of your gown, keep in mind that light complexions work better with the darker whites. A bright white will cause a light complexion to wash out, especially if the gown has a glossy sheen under bright light. If you have a light complexion and have your heart set on a bright white dress, you should choose a fabric with a matte sheen to improve the contrast.

Likewise, darker complexions work best with the brighter whites. If you have a dark complexion and your heart is set on one of the darker white colors, you should choose a glossy sheen to create the needed contrast. In any event, choose a color that compliments your complexion.

This brings up the topic of undertones. Skin is made up of a lot of colors, and these colors need to be considered when you select your gown. The basic undertones are yellow/orange, orange/red, red, and blue/red. All of these undertones can exist despite your actual primary skin color, although every primary skin color will favor a particular undertone. African American skin tones tend to favor red, yellow, blue, and orange. The fairer Latino skin tones lean toward orange, red, and yellow. The lighter Asians tend to favor yellows, while the light Caucasian skin tones favor red. As you choose your gown and accessory colors (especially your flowers), you should consider the undertone of your skin.

FITTING YOUR DRESS

Once you've determined the style of your gown, it's time to concentrate on the fit. Most bridal salons carry an array of sample gown sizes for determining what size should be ordered. Until recently, the largest sample in most salons was a 14 or—if you were lucky—a 16. Thankfully, many shops now have samples up to a size 20. If you need a larger size, be sure to call ahead to find out if they carry it. Don't fret if they say no; a creative bridal consultant can work magic.

You must, however, do your part to make sure the right size is ordered. Be sure you take the following items with you to your fitting:

Shoes These should have heels the same height as the shoes you will be wearing on your wedding day. (Make sure you select a comfortable pair. You'll be in them a long time.)

Bridal Undergarments Bridal gowns require far more than your average bra, panty, and slip combination. The next section will help you select the best type of undergarments for your dress style. However, if you haven't purchased them by the time you try on your gown, or if you are still debating between styles, some salons have bridal slips you can use.

Now that you're dressed in a gown, here's what you need to do:

- Raise your arms and move them around. See how you feel if your dress has the following attributes:

  Strapless bodice: Is the dress comfortable under your collarbone and across the back? Is the material so tight that it chaffs your skin? Is there a gap? Are you at risk for an embarrassing moment?

  Sleeveless: Can you move your arms comfortably? Does the material pull when moved, or is there too much of a gap? Can you raise your arms without taking the whole bodice with you? If you lean over, does the armhole stay in place or does it gap open?

  Long-Sleeved: Do the sleeves feel confining? Is it tight along the shoulder line? Are the sleeves too big? Can you move your arms without pulling the material?

  Short-Sleeved: Do the tops of the sleeves drape comfortably over your shoulders? Are the sleeves tight around your upper arms? Can you move your arms around with confidence?

  Spaghetti Straps: Do the straps dig into your skin? Do the straps keep falling down, no matter how you move?

- Now consider the waist and bodice. There are a number of different bodices, but the same rules apply. Does the material pull around your waist? Can you sit down comfortably?

  What about breathing? Do you feel constricted when you're standing? How about when you sit? Remember, the idea is to leave *him* breathless, not you.

- And now the skirt. Walk around the dressing room with your shoes on. Do you feel like you're going to trip? Does the material feel too heavy to carry as you walk? Can you sit down?

  Is the material too stiff to make a bathroom visit possible during the reception? Does the material move with you as you walk, or does it seem to work against you?

- Since you are likely to have at least one friend with you, ask her to be your partner and pretend you're dancing your first dance. How does the gown feel overall? Are there any little nuisances—like a button that pulls or an edge that doesn't stay in place? Will your groom be able to hold you tight? Or can he reach you through the tulle?

Take a look in the mirror. These are the moments of your life that will be immortalized on film. Be sure your smile is natural. There is nothing worse on film than a forced grin caused by an ill-fitting gown. Be honest. Your wedding is supposed to be a day to enjoy. You don't want to spend it constantly distracted because you're uncomfortable.

CUSTOM GOWNS

Suppose the adventure of shopping around becomes too much, or you simply can't find what you are looking for? A possible alternative is to find a designer to help you bring your vision to reality.

Should this be the case, you will need to budget an additional three to six months to accommodate the custom gown process. That means you will need to begin at least a year or more in advance of your wedding date to plan your entire wedding.

Check around for qualified designers or seamstresses in your area. Get recommendations and schedule an appointment to meet with one of them. I strongly recommend working with a professional. While it might be convenient to have a friend or relative sew the dress, what will your recourse be if he or she suddenly takes ill or has a family emergency? By engaging a professional, you have the added insurance of a contractual obligation that your gown will be finished in time for your wedding.

A Checklist for the Designer or Seamstress

1. Bring photos or ads of dress styles you like.

2. If you find a dress pattern you like, bring it or the pattern number with you to the appointment.

3. Regardless of whether you use a pattern or have an original design made, be sure to discuss which areas of your figure you would like to play up and those you want toned down. Also remember to discuss any personal touches you may want added, such as a family crest or design relevant to your cultural heritage.

4. Ask if the designer does muslin gown samples. Many designers and seamstresses use muslin during the design process to get an idea of how the finished dress will look. If they do make samples, ask if they use plus-size mannequins.

5. Give the designer your budget and ask for fabric suggestions. If you already have a fabric in mind, are they willing to allow you to purchase it yourself? Or will they make the purchase?

6. Verify the approximate number of fittings you will need to schedule to accommodate any changes (for weight loss, etc.).

7. Don't forget to ask how many dresses they do per week/month/quarter, etc. This will help you de-

termine how quickly they can produce your dress, and also let you know how much experience they have had. Ask to see their portfolio.

8. Ask to see a sample of their contract. Are they willing to provide you with client references? What is their payment and refund policy?

9. If at any time during the process you are not satisfied with the gown, can you make changes or alterations?

10. Do they make headpieces? Or can they recommend someone who does?

11. When the dress is finished, will they press or steam it there? Or do you have to take it to the cleaners?

12. Most importantly, find out how long the process will take from start to finish.

Having a gown made can be a wonderful option. If you find the right person to work with, the results will be simply beautiful.

UNDERGARMENTS

We've talked about the outside; now we need to get down to the nuts and bolts that hold your whole look together—the undergarments.

Bridal lingerie is a broad term that refers to everything from bikinis to nightgowns. Bridal undergarments, on the other hand, are the functional foundation garments—bras, bustiers, and body shapers—that keep everything in place and looking perfect under your gown. Bridal undergarments also include an assortment of slips designed specifically to give gowns the right look.

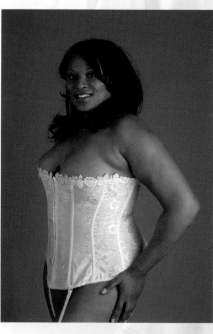

Though the word "foundation" seems a bit old-fashioned, it is accurate. Before you slip on the dress of your dreams, you need to have the appropriate foundation on which to build your "brick house." Am I saying we need control garments because of our size? Absolutely not. What I am saying is that they can help build a better "bombshell" by making those curves even curvier.

Now before you panic, please realize that undergarments have come a long way from your grandmother's (or even your mother's) day. Today's designs afford control without pain. And not only are they more comfortable, they can actually be called sexy.

Full-figure lingerie has also come a long way. We now have options like sexy bikinis, French cuts, thongs, and for the truly daring, G-strings. And while tradition dictates that your undergarments be as white and demure as you are, that doesn't mean you can't add your own spicy touches to your "demure" ensemble. If you choose to wear something a bit daring underneath it all, well, that's your secret—and his. How about a lace bikini as your "something blue"!

Upper Body Undergarments

But back to the basics. As with any other part of your clothing, getting the correct size in undergarments is vital to really looking good.

Think you know your bra size by now? Chances are you don't, and you're not alone. Over 60% of us are wearing the wrong size bra right now. Pay a visit to your local lingerie boutique and get measured by a professional. A properly fitted bra alleviates bulges, excess "unfilled" cups, slipping up in back, and other traditional bra complaints.

Now with regard to your gown, all upper body undergarments—strapless, bustier, corset, demi, miracle, or full coverage—do the same thing: they keep you supported. Any of them will do the job. Just choose the one that fits your gown's bodice style and your personal preference.

For strapless gowns, the best choice is a merry widow or bustier with extra boning in the bodice and cup. The fit should be snug but not uncomfortable. When you try on a bustier, take several different sizes into the dressing room with you; then, as you try each one, move around to see if it pokes into your skin. Make sure you have enough room to breathe, but be careful not to choose one so large that you risk falling out of your dress!

Gowns with sleeves and/or wide straps allow for versatility. Either a bustier or a traditional bra will suit them equally well. Again, be sure of the fit. Move around. Is anything poking or pinching? Make sure the straps are sturdy enough to support you, but not digging into your shoulders. And once you have your undergarments and your gown on together, make sure the straps are concealed by the gown.

If you are considering a backless gown, you may want to try disposable, self-adhesive crescents. These little wonders actually go from size A to size DD. For larger bust sizes, use two for each breast. They are strapless, sideless, and backless, and they last for up to 12 hours. They can, however, be hard to find outside of lingerie catalogs or on-line shops, so plan ahead and allow plenty of time for delivery.

As a side note, while all of these options may apply equally well to bridesmaids, wearing a bustier or corset may prove to be a bit much for them. After all, they're not the one in the spotlight. As an alternative, consider an adjustable bra such as Lane Bryant's 5-way with seamless underwire support. It is economical, much less restrictive, and it will be useful far beyond the wedding.

Body Suits

For sheath gowns, I recommend a body suit to keep the line of the dress smooth. Body slips tend to keep riding up no matter what you do, but a body suit will stay in place and it comes in full coverage, French cut, or thong styles. It also brings us to the lower half of the undergarment world.

Just as your upper body foundation is based on the neckline of your gown, the shaper or slimmer you choose is determined by your gown's waistline and skirt. Formfitting gowns such as a sheath, column, or mermaid demand a one piece foundation garment. Other waist and skirt styles let you base your decision strictly on your personal preference.

A word about quality and care . . . before you plop down your money, make sure the construction of an undergarment is sturdy. Does the material snap back into place when you pull it? Is it sheer or flimsy? Are there any snags in the material that might unravel at the worst possible moment? Look at the underwire. Is it double stitched to prevent it from poking out? Is the garment sturdy enough to do the job for which you are buying it? Remember, you're spending your hard earned dollars, and bridal lingerie does have a life after the wedding, so be sure you get something that will last. Then remember to hand wash your garments after you've worn them. Machine washing may be tempting, but it will ruin the garment's shape and decrease its shelf life. If you do machine wash, use the gentle cycle and a mild detergent such as Woolite or Ivory Snow.

Slips

The final consideration for your undergarments is the bridal slip. A bridal slip is more than just a standard slip. An everyday slip gives a dress body and helps it flow gracefully as you move. A bridal slip goes one step further. It adds fullness to the gown's skirt, and it is built to support the weight and sheer volume of the cloth involved in a full gown. While a regular full-length slip may be sufficient for fitted styles, full gowns need an appropriate bridal slip to give them their intended look. The last thing you want is to spend money on the dress of your dreams only to have it fall flat.

Bridal slips are categorized by how full they are. Medium and medium-full slips are the most common choice since they accommodate the largest number of gowns. They are well suited to column and A-line gowns. If your gown needs more lift to achieve the look you want, move to a full slip. Extra full and hoop slips are for dramatic sweeping effects, such as with a gown that has a ball silhouette.

There is one distinct difference between a hoop slip and other bridal slips: the hoop relies on boning or wire to hold its flared shape. This causes the slip to flare at or near the waist, and gives the gown a "Scarlet O'Hara" look. By comparison, an extra full slip lets a gown fall in gathers, flaring more toward the hemline. A dramatic example of this would be a trumpet style skirt.

It is worth noting that, as with all things, bridal terminology tends to vary both by region and with time. Companies want to make their products sound new and exciting to entice buyers, and the result is often confusion for the customer. If you find yourself in this situation, don't be afraid to go with your own intuition. Try on different slips with the gown you like, and take the one that best suits your taste and the design of your dress.

Consultants and Shops

Some bridal consultants will be able to assist you with your undergarment choices; however, most are unfamiliar with the types of garments available. This is where a specialty shop comes in handy. Lingerie specialty shops and websites know everything there is to know about undergarments and can be quite helpful. Some bridal shops and chains will refer brides to local shops or websites. (And of course you can't beat word-of-mouth.)

A number of lingerie shops and chains carry bridal lingerie; as noted earlier, however, there is a slight difference between bridal lingerie and bridal undergarments. While bridal lingerie often refers to bras, panties, bustiers, hosiery, body slimmers and garter belts, it also refers to teddies, peignoirs, and nightgowns. The term bridal undergarments refers exclusively to foundation garments: bras, bustiers, merry widows, body slimmers (shapers) and slips (petticoats).

Using the yellow pages, look under bridal salons and lingerie shops/boutiques. (NOTE: when looking under either heading, be sure to call the shop to see if they carry the type of undergarments a bride needs.) To look up online resources, bring up a search engine (Google, Yahoo, Lycos, etc.) and type in "bridal undergarments," "bridal slips," "bridal accessories," or "bridal foundation garments."

JEWELRY

The choice of wedding jewelry—beyond the engagement and wedding ring—is another important element of your bridal ensemble. There are various styles of necklaces to choose from, as well as a wide variety of earrings and bracelets. Necklaces can be broadly categorized into three styles: chokers (one fitted strand or strap worn close to the neck); collars (several strands that fit securely around the base of the neck); or T-style (a princess [hanging strand] necklace with a dangling strand hanging down from the bottom of the necklace, generally forming a "T" design).

Chokers are worn high on the neck to emphasize the neck. Collar necklaces are worn at the base of the neck and emphasize the shoulders and bosom. The T-style or princess necklace is the most common style of the three. It can range in length from 14–19 inches, although the most common length is 17–19 inches. It is perfect for high necklines. Its length falls below the hollow of the neck in front, providing perfect support for a pendant.

Earrings should match the metals and jewels of your necklace, but their design will be dictated by the shape of your face. An oval- or diamond-shaped face can use button, round, or hoop earrings. Triangular earrings are especially flattering. Dangling earrings work well if they aren't too long.

On a round face, square, oblong, or rectangle earrings work well. Also, angular and dangling styles look nice, especially for plus-size brides. The elongated styles will draw attention down, giving the face a thinner appearance.

A rectangular or oblong face needs earrings that add width, making the face appear shorter, while a heart-shaped face looks good in earrings that are wider at the bottom than at the top. Earrings that form a triangle and dangle can be especially flattering.

Keep in mind that if your dress is very plain, a more decorative earring will work well. If your dress is very ornate, however, a plainer design would work best. You want to compliment—not detract—from the design of your dress.

Bracelets may not be an option if you are wearing gloves or have long sleeves, especially sleeves with decorative cuffs. However, if your dress is strapless, or you are using a shorter sleeve and are not wearing gloves, you may want to choose an unobtrusive bracelet that matches the style of your necklace and earrings.

Although the jewels and metals you select are a personal choice, there are some considerations that go beyond the type of gown you've chosen. We have already determined the role body type plays in choosing a gown. The same applies to jewelry choices, especially necklaces. Remember—it is important to select a necklace made to fit a fuller figure; in other words, not all chokers are created equal. For inverted triangle and round body shapes, necklace choices should draw the eye's attention downward, thereby elongating the neck and upper body. For this reason, collars and chokers should be avoided. For rectangle, diamond, and pear shapes—where the shoulders are narrow—the necklace should draw the eye up toward the shoulders. Collars and chokers work well on these body types. For hourglass shapes, any type of necklace can be worn since the upper and lower body is equally balanced.

You also need to consider the shape of your face when you select your necklace. The following list indicates what works well with the various face shapes:

Oval/Diamond/ These are the most flexible face shapes and provide the most options for jewelry. All styles
Oblong Face can be worn as long as they work well with the style of the bride's gown.

Round Face Use a longer or T-style necklace and look for smaller stones because large stones will draw negative attention to the neck. Avoid chokers and collars. Collars tend to make the neck area appear larger. Chokers (especially wide chokers,) make the face and neck appear wider. They also give the neck a constricted look.

Heart-Shaped Face Chokers and collars work to add depth to the narrowness of the chin and create a full look around the neck area.

Square Face Use a T-style (princess or hanging strand) necklace.

Rectangle Face Rectangle shapes need width, so short necklaces, collars, and chokers work well.

Triangle Face To soften the angular edges, stay away from necklaces that come to a point.

CASUAL WEAR

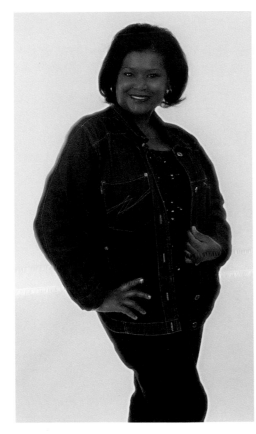

Even though this guide is all about bridal styles, you're going to need clothes to wear besides the wedding gown. The same concepts that make you look your best in your wedding gown will also make you look great in a blouse or a sweater. After all, you have to have something comfortable, fashionable, and stylish while you go shopping, right?

At one time, plus-size women had few options when it came to finding fashionable casual wear. Most styles were as big, boxy, and shapeless as designers thought full-figured women were. Thankfully, times have changed. Now there are as many styles and options as there are designers. Here are two that you might not have considered as fashionable:

Jeans

Denim is as American as apple pie, but for many years, finding a pair of jeans that actually fit was like trying to find the proverbial needle in a haystack. Fortunately, this is no longer the case. Gambino Jeans, Venezia, Avenue Blues, and Ashley Stewart (just to name a few) design fashionable jeans to fit the curves of full-figured women of every shape and height. Moreover, the designs are trendy, sexy, fashionable, and definitely not your "grandfather's" jeans.

Workout/Spa/Yoga Wear

Another option for comfort and style is that of workout wear. I'm not talking about shapeless sweat suits, but sleek styles that easily go from the gym to the mall and still look good.

Yoga wear is especially popular today as many people are turning to yoga to find their chakras and align them with the universe. Whether or not you embrace the idea of yoga, you can embrace the clothes. Fashion Bug Plus, Just My Size, and Delta Burke are some of the designers who design sensible and practical workout wear for full-figured women: i.e., workout tops with built-in shelf bras for support.

WHAT TO WEAR AFTER THE RECEPTION

While it is important to concentrate on what to wear for your wedding, it is equally important to think about what you'll wear after the reception when you make your getaway. This decision depends on a few factors:

- What time of day is your reception? If you get married in the afternoon, you'll either be leaving your reception to head directly to your honeymoon destination, or staying overnight at a hotel to depart the next day.

- The reception location. If you get married in a hotel, chances are you will have a bridal or honeymoon suite reserved as a part of your wedding package—so your groom can carry you over the threshold in your gown.

The most important factor to consider is that there are no hard and fast rules as to what you must wear after the reception. It's all a matter of taste. You can wear a suit, pants suit, dress, gown, or even jeans if you want. It all depends on you, so suit yourself.

Beautiful Women

Hair, makeup, and accessories all play a very important part in your overall wedding style. This is the time to look your best, and all of these elements will play a pivotal role in both how you are seen and how you see yourself.

HAIR

There is no doubt in my mind that all brides make time to get their hair done. No matter how you normally wear your hair, you are going to want something special for your wedding day. Of course, how you wear your hair is your own personal choice, but you want to be sure that it makes a statement about you.

Choosing the right hairstyle is a very important decision. There are many elements to consider, not the least of which is your opinion of what looks good on you. However, you must be mindful of the shape of your face and the type of hair you have in order to choose the most flattering style.

As noted, faces can be grouped into eight general shapes: oval, round, oblong, heart (inverted triangle), square, rectangle, diamond, and triangle. If you are in doubt as to which shape you have, take these measurements: your face across the top of your cheekbones; your jawline between the widest points; your forehead at its widest point; and from your hairline to the bottom of your chin. Write each of these measurements down. Round faces and square faces are approximately as long as they are wide. With an oval face, the length of the face will equal one and one-half times its width. An oblong face will be longer than it is wide with the forehead, cheekbones, and brow bones being about the same width. A rectangular face is long and narrow with cheeks that appear to be hollow. A diamond-shaped face will be narrow through the forehead and chin, but wider through the cheekbones. A heart-shaped/inverted triangle face will be wide at the temples and hairline, narrowing to a small delicate chin. Finally, a triangle shape will be the reverse of the heart shape, with a dominant jawline and a narrowing at the cheekbones, temple, and forehead.

Next, ask yourself what type of hair you have. Is it straight, curly, kinky, or wavy? What about texture? Is it "polyester" fine, medium, or silky rope thick? And consider volume. The more hairs per square inch, the greater the volume.

Face shapes
Now let's find the most flattering style for you:

Oval Face

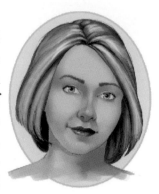

Lucky lady. The oval face is generally wider at the temples than at the jawline and has a gently rounded hairline. Women with oval faces have a great deal of latitude in the hair styles they can choose. It is a shape commonly found on models. You can wear your hair short, medium, or long with this shape depending on the texture of your hair. However, it is wise to avoid heavy bangs or bringing too much hair onto the face, since the spatial planes of an oval face tend to be smaller than other shapes.

You will recognize many of the well-know personalities who have oval-shaped faces, among them Cameron Diaz, Mariah Carey, Julia Roberts, Heather Locklear, and Cindy Crawford.

Round Face

If your face is round and full with the widest point at the cheeks and ears, try one of the following:

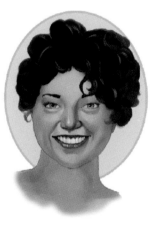

- Off-center parts are flattering.

- A full hairstyle with height at the crown works well with medium and fine hair.

- Longer hairstyles that fall below the chin level work well with heavy, straight hair.

- A short hairstyle brushed away from the face is especially good for fine, curly hair.

- A variety of hair types can layer the hair on top of the head to create fullness while cutting the rest fairly close to the face.

All of these styles are designed to make the round face appear narrower and a little longer. Because the widest part of your face is at the cheeks and ears, you need to avoid styles that create fullness in those areas. You also want to avoid hair styles that have center parts or straight bangs, that are cropped very short, or that hang cup-like around the circular shape of the head and end below the ears. These all accentuate the fullness of a round face. Actresses Drew Barrymore and Roseanne Barr are examples of women with round faces.

Oblong Face

The forehead, cheekbones, and brow bones are thin and of equal width on an oblong face. It is generally best to balance this shape with short to medium length layered hair styles that have full sides. The hair should be parted off-center for longer styles. Stay away from center parts; they will make the face seem longer. Take a tip from Julia Ormond. With longer styles, she avoids a distinct part and draws a loose bang over her forehead to offset the length of her face.

Heart-shaped Face

If your face is heart-shaped, it will be wide at the temples and hairline with a small chin. The following styles look great:

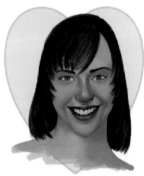

- Styles that are chin length or longer and add fullness to the lower face.

- Styles that use a side part.

- Swept forward layers around the upper face.

- Soft bangs to de-emphasize the width of the forehead.

- Shorter styles that leave a little weight in the back nape area.

It would be wise to avoid short, full styles that emphasize the upper face. They will make you look top heavy. Other no-no's include: styles that are high at the crown; styles that have a slicked back look; or short, full styles with a tapered neckline. These tend to emphasize the upper face. Instead, emphasize your cheekbones. Michelle Pfeiffer and Ashley Judd have learned how to do it.

Square Face

Square-shaped faces have strong jawlines and broad foreheads. Try some of the following:

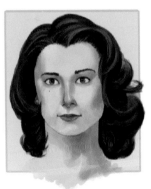

- Off-center parts.

- Height at the crown with wispy bangs.

- Short to medium length hair, especially if it waves or seems to round or soften the square corners of the face.

- Curly layers around the face.

The objective is to soften the square look of the face. Avoid styles that are linear, such as straight bangs or center parts. Long, straight styles will emphasize a square jawbone. You want to produce roundness and height. Sandra Bullock and Demi Moore both have square faces. Take a cue from their hairstyles.

Rectangular Face

Rectangular faces are long and slender with the same width at the forehead as at the cheekbones. They commonly have high foreheads or a narrow chin. Some of the best styles for this shape of face are:

- Short to medium lengths that produce fullness at the sides of the head. This balances the long appearance of the face.

- Soft bangs to shorten the appearance of length.

- Layers to soften the straight lines of the rectangular face.

Avoid wearing your hair too long or too high—it will make your face look even longer. Go for the soft, feminine look, like Kirstie Alley and Gwyneth Paltrow.

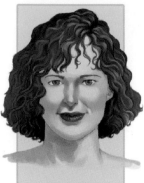

Diamond-shaped Face

The diamond shape is characterized by a narrow forehead and chin with wide cheek bones. Choose hair styles that frame the face, but keep the sides close to the face to avoid making it appear wider. It is flattering to promote height at the crown of the head and add fullness below the chin. The goal is to create an oval appearance and lift the facial features. Elizabeth Hurley's hair style is a good example. You can also see the results on such actresses as Sophia Loren and Katherine Hepburn: both classic, beautiful ladies.

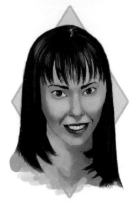

Triangular Face

Use short, layered hair styles that emphasize fullness around the temple area to bring balance to the jawline. Stay away from chin length styles that make that zone appear more pronounced. Long hair can be styled to draw attention to the temple area with a side part. Hairstyles for a triangular face should be just the reverse of those for a heart-shaped face. Off-center parts, wedges, and shags look great on these ladies. Just avoid anything that draws attention to the jawline. See how Kathy Ireland does it.

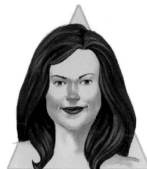

Hair Color

Every now and then, a girl likes to spice up her life and her attitude by adding a little color to her hair. For many of us, it is an inexpensive form of therapy that will give our spirits a lift. But before you go from a brunette to a platinum blonde, you need to remember that what you see on the box is not always what you get. It will vary with your natural hair color. Most hair color products have a chart on the back that can give you a rough idea of how you will look based on your starting color.

Before you pick out a color, you should be mindful of your natural skin tone. The colors that work well for different skin tones will generally fall into two categories (although there are exceptions):

Cool colors: Fair to light, medium, and olive skin tones
Warm colors: Fair to medium brown, bronze and mocha skin tones

According to Clairol, complementary cool colors will have the words "ash" or "neutral" in their descriptors. Complementary warm colors will have the words "warm" or "reddish" in their descriptors. For more information on hair color, check out www.clairol.com.

Although there are a number of reasonably priced and relatively easy do-it-yourself hair color kits available, I strongly recommend that you seek the services of a hair professional. Professional hair stylists are trained to handle chemical color processes with less room for error. Unless your best friend or your Aunt Mary is a beautician, resist the urge to do it yourself. Not only will you save your hair, you will save yourself a very big headache. I can't emphasize this enough—don't do it yourself!

Now, let me offer a word of caution about making any major changes. Don't do it a week before the wedding. According to Ronice Davis of Sittin' Pretty, "Try a new color long before the wedding; as far as six months in advance is optimal."

Hair Care

Healthy hair is the result of a good diet, consistently diligent maintenance, and most important, the right hair care professional. If you don't already have a regular stylist, you should find one at least eight months to a year before the big day. According to T.J. and Taschia of the House of Essence in Amityville, New York, "A beautician needs to get to know you and your hair's special needs." A good stylist will base his or her recommendations and treatment on six basic factors:

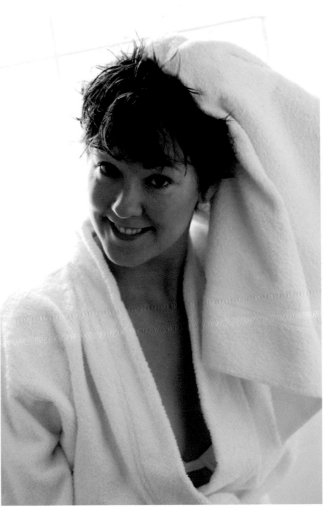

1. The condition of your hair—is it damaged, weak, overprocessed, oily, dry, etc.

2. Any scalp conditions, such as dandruff, eczema, or psoriasis.

3. The consistency of your hair: fine, superfine, curly, wavy, or coarse.

4. Whether your hair is chemically treated with a perm, a relaxer, and/or color.

5. Whether you are taking medications that can affect your hair, such as birth control pills, medication for blood pressure, diabetes, epilepsy, or MS, etc.

6. External stress factors such as job changes, moving, and—planning a wedding!

All of these factors play a role in determining the best course of treatment for your hair. Once you've begun a treatment course with a stylist, T.J. and Taschia recommend a visit to the beauty salon on either a weekly or bi-weekly basis. However, if you aren't able to keep up with that schedule, there are things you can do in order to maintain your hair's healthy balance.

- Choose a shampoo according to your hair type. If you have color treated hair, use a shampoo made for color treated hair. If you have a scalp condition, i.e., dandruff, etc., use a shampoo formulated for dandruff or any other problem your hair may have.

- Shampoo regularly, and always follow with a good conditioning treatment suitable for your hair type and condition (read the labels). Although shampooing rids hair of dirt and deposits, it strips away natural hair oils that need to be replenished. (If your hair is chemically treated or relaxed, consider using a conditioning rinse or semi-permanent color to avoid damage.)

- Don't be afraid to get a professional trim every six to eight weeks to remove split ends and over-processed hair. You may need a trim more often if you wear your hair short. Of, if you are trying to grow your hair out, every 12–13 weeks.

- If you have always sworn your hair long and you want a drastic change, be sure you are ready to part with it before the first snip. A few tears during the ceremony are sweet. Full-blown weeping and sobbing are a bit less demure.

- Don't use heated styling products more than once a week. Use pin curls, wraps, and rollers to help maintain curls or shape.

- When buying blow dryers, flat irons, and curling irons, look for products with ceramic heat and low electromagnetic fields (EMF). It's more moisturizing and better for you.

- Do not attempt to do any chemical treatments at home. Hair stylists are trained to handle the mixing and application of hair chemicals without causing damage. (For chemically relaxed hair, T.J. recommends skipping at least one relaxer for more noticeable hair growth.)

Tips for Choosing the Right Salon

1. Ask your friends, family, or co-workers for recommendations, then schedule an interview. Most salons want your business and will accommodate you. Take a little notepad and jot down some general and specific questions to pose.

2. Check out the atmosphere. Is it a calm, relaxing place—or does it seem more like an assembly line? Do they take a full client history of your hair and overall health? Do they keep client profile sheets on file in the establishment to review for every appointment?

3. Do they discuss hair style options and services with clients to determine whether a particular style is a viable option, or are they more concerned with the bottom line (money)?

How can a stylist make a difference? Here is an example. According to Taschia, many clients request that hair extensions or weaves be a part of their bridal look. While she is happy to oblige her clients with what they want, she is careful to note the amount of time and care required to maintain the extensions on the honeymoon. In order to bring this point home, she will occasionally give a client a "test run weave" before the wedding. In most cases, the bride-to-be recognizes the work involved in taking care of a weave in her everyday life, and realizes it doesn't fit into honeymoon fun. However, Taschia notes this is a matter of personal taste. Brides who are planning to lie on the beach or by the pool will be able to keep their extensions/weaves in place. But if a bride is planning to surf, scuba dive, go skiing, or participate in any of the more active sports, hair extensions/weaves may not be the wisest choice.

Again, this demonstrates the importance of having a relationship with your stylist. She can help guard you against making bad hair decisions while still keeping you firmly in the driver's seat. In other words, if you like your hair long, wear it long. If you want to wear an upsweep, wear it. Love your hair short? Cut it. Want highlights? Highlight away. But work with your stylist to indulge yourself within the framework of what looks good on you based on the shape of your face and the type of hair you have.

You get the picture.

Also, don't forget to bring a friend or two along for their input. Better yet, bring your bridesmaids along for their wedding day hairstyles. This way you can bond and have fun while you make yourselves beautiful.

If you've decided on a headpiece, bring it with you to see how your vision will look as a total picture. This trial run is a perfect opportunity to work out all the kinks so that styling your hair for your wedding day will be relaxing and effortless.

Dos and Don'ts

Here's a quick summary to guide you as you get ready to decide on your wedding day do:

Hairstyle Dos:

*   Visit your salon to establish a hair care plan at least six to eight months before the wedding.
*   Regularly wash and condition your hair.
*   Use a deep conditioner.
*   Get your hair trimmed every six to eight weeks to combat split ends.
*   Schedule your final trim two weeks before the wedding.
*   If you color your hair, touch it up two weeks prior to the wedding.

HAIR

- Pay extra attention to your ends, and wrap your hair before going to bed to prevent breakage.

- Decide whether or not you will be removing your veil once the ceremony is over. This will affect the hairstyle you choose.

- Make sure your hairdo is weatherproof if you are planning an outdoor wedding.

Hairstyle Don'ts:

- Don't make any major hair changes right before the wedding.

- Don't experiment with new hair products too close to your wedding day in case of an allergic reaction.

- Don't style your hair too early on your wedding day.

- Don't over-condition your hair, it will weigh it down.

Follow this simple advice for a more beautiful, happy you on your wedding (or any other) day.

SKIN CARE

As with any artist, you need a clean canvas on which to create a masterpiece. Good basic skin care is the key to nearly flawless makeup. So if you don't know your skin type by now, you should make it a priority to find out.

Skin Type

The following are some guidelines to help you determine which skin type you have, and how you should care for it.

Normal Skin

Normal skin is the goal of every skin care program. The skin is soft, smooth, and firm, and blemishes are uncommon. The pores are small to medium in size. The skin is evenly toned and balanced. Normal skin has good elasticity and is smooth and firm to the touch. However, even normal skin will have some oily areas. The term "T-zone" refers to an area that stretches across the forehead and down the nose and chin. This is the area that occasionally presents problems.

When cleansing this skin type, use products that keep the skin hydrated. Use a water-based moisturizer, although you should apply it less frequently to the oily areas of the face. Products that contain alpha hydroxyl acids and vitamin A retinols work well to help maintain balance in skin tone. Some products of this type that can be found in department stores are Lancôme's Gel Clarté, Tonique Clarté, Exfoliance Clarté, and Pure Focus Lotion; also Iman's Liquid Assets Gentle Cleansing Lotion. There are also some very good moisturizers and cleansers to be found in your local drugstore, such as Oil of Olay's Daily Care Active Hydrating Cream and Daily Facials Express for all skin types. I use their moisturizer for sensitive skin with SPF protection. To reduce shine, use oil absorbing makeup.

Oily Skin

Oily skin is shiny in appearance with more noticeable pores that are medium to large in size. Problems include clogged pores, blackheads, whiteheads and blemishes.

To be sure your face is at its best, develop a routine to cleanse your skin regularly using a soap-free face wash that rinses easily. Use a mild toner after cleansing, while your pores are open. However, be sure the toner is not alcohol-based; alcohol irritates the skin and could damage it. I recommend using any of the following: Lancôme's Pure Focus Cleanser and Pure Focus Toner, or Prescriptives' All Clean Sparkling Gel Cleanser and Immediate Matte Skin Conditioning Tonic for Normal/Oilier Skin. These are available at many department stores. From the drugstore, Oil of Olay's Daily Facials Clarity Toner and Ponds' Cool Calm & Perfected Pore-Shrinking Toner are great for all skin types.

Having pore trouble? The funny thing about pores is that they are often big enough to hold blackheads, but small enough to make it impossible to get rid of blackheads without visiting a dermatologist on a regular basis. I remember my mother contorting my nose and cheeks trying to get my pores to release the offenders. Ouch!

Thankfully, we now have products to clean pores without pain. Both Ponds and Bioré make nose strips (and now even facial strips) to lift both blackheads and whiteheads away. While these products don't leave the same type of redness my mother left on my face, they can still cause minor irritation. Therefore, in order to maximize the benefits, try to use them at least two to three days before the wedding to make sure any redness dissipates.

Dry Skin

If your skin feels tight on your face, flakes off, is easily irritated, or is sensitive to cold weather, you probably have dry skin. The dryness is caused by the loss of moisture (not oil). If you normally don't feel that your skin is dry, environmental factors may be the cause. You may not be drinking enough water, or you may be affected by certain types of heating in the winter or by being in the wind for prolonged periods of time.

Inappropriate skin care routines can also cause dry skin, such as the use of harsh cleansers, or not following up with a moisturizer for protection. Be sure to use an oil free, non-comedogenic (won't clog pores) moisturizer. Try Clinique's Dramatically Different Moisturizing Lotion or Clinique's Superdefense Triple

Action Moisturizer with SPF 25 for very dry skin. Oil of Olay's Complete Defense Daily UV Moisturizer with SPF 30 also works well.

If you have recently changed soaps, that could be another factor. Soaps in general tend to be drying, and those with added moisturizers can cause allergic reactions. If you have changed cleansing products lately and are experiencing a difference in skin tone, you may need to change again.

It is difficult to diagnose the reason for dry skin for any given person due to the many factors that can cause it. To further complicate the process, certain medications and medical conditions such as diabetes can also affect your skin. Therefore, the best plan of action is to consistently use soap-free cleansers, and avoid products containing mineral oil, petroleum, lanolin, alcohol, artificial colors, and fragrances. Try Lancôme's Gel Clarté, Tonique Clarté, or Exfoliance Clarté; Clinique's Clarifying Lotion or Clarifying Lotion 2; Neutrogena's Extra Gentle Cleanser; or Ponds' Fresh Start Cleanser.

Combination Skin

Combination skin is like having a split personality. One part may be dry while another is oily. The T-zone areas are oily while the cheeks and the areas around the eyes are either normal or dry. This condition describes the majority of combination skin types, except for a small percentage of women who may have such symptoms as a pimply forehead or oily cheeks while all else is normal. The skin may be normal everywhere outside the T-zone, but this would still be considered a combination skin type.

Be careful not to over wash your face. This will only exacerbate this condition by stripping the oil from the T-zone, causing the sebaceous glands to produce more sebum to compensate. Look for cleansers suitable for combination skin. A deep-pore cleanser will help keep the oily T-zone clear. A non-comedogenic moisturizer will provide enough hydration without making the oilier areas worse. If you think this isn't enough for you, try a moisturizer made with light silicone oils. They don't cause excessive oiliness. Some excellent products of this type are Lancôme's Aqua Fusion Lotion, Lancôme's Bienfait Multi-Vital SPF 30 Lotion, Iman's Perfect Response Oil Free Hydrating Gel, or Oil of Olay's Complete All Day Moisture Lotion with SPF 15. A mild toner will help to keep skin shine-free in the T-zone. However, it is not necessary for the drier zones.

When you exfoliate, pay special attention to oilier areas such as the chin, nose and forehead. A gel mask suits combination skin. Or try using two different masks: a clay mask for the oil-prone nose, chin, and forehead, and a cream mask for dry areas, such as the cheeks. I recommend Clinique's Total Turnaround Visible Skin Renewer, Lancôme's Rénergie Intense Lift Mask, Lancôme's Pure Empreinte Masque Purifying Mineral Mask with White Clay, and Neutrogena's Deep Clean Oil-Controlling Mask.

Sensitive Skin

People with sensitive skin have a lot more trouble with environmental factors than the average person. Their skin burns more easily in the sun, they have more sensitivity to cosmetics (particularly if perfumed), and they may experience rashes or a burning sensation when overexposed to wind, sun, and extreme shifts in temperature. If your skin is easily irritated, you may be a sensitive skin type. Look for soap, makeup, and moisturizers that are fragrance-free and hypoallergenic. Some good products are Prescriptives' Comfort Cleanser Gentle Lotion for Sensitive Skin; Prescriptives' Comfort Lotion, Oil Free for Sensitive Skin; Oil of Olay's Daily Facials Cleansing Cloths (soothing for sensitive skin); and Ponds' Pristine Clean Gentle Cleansing Foam for sensitive skin. Wash your face once a day and avoid using skin exfoliants. Use a hypoallergenic toner on oily areas, such as Ponds' Cool, Calm & Perfected Pore-Shrinking Gel Toner for all skin types, or Estée Lauder's Vérité Soothing Spray Toner. However, discontinue their use if they cause irritation.

It is not necessary to invade the counters of department stores when you do begin looking for a skin care system. There are many smaller retailers that cater to skin and makeup products. Or a visit to the skin care aisle in your local pharmacy can provide a number of choices that do the same job without all the overhead of a department or specialty store. Find a product that best suits your needs and lifestyle.

If you already have a skin care system that works for you, stick with it. Do not change your skin care system dramatically before the wedding. The stress of planning your wedding with all its day-to-day pressures is a recipe for more breakouts. The key here is to compensate by cleansing, exfoliating, and moisturizing your skin. If you have a system you've been using for a while, chances are any additional breakouts can be handled with an increase in toner or a decrease in moisturizer.

If you don't follow a skin care regimen, your wedding provides a great excuse to begin. Many biohazards (such as pollution) have been known to affect skin. Our skin is our largest organ, and it is on the front lines in the war against pollutants and the decreasing ozone layer. Even those of us with more melanin have to protect our skin from the sun's cancer-causing rays. Skin cancer was once thought of as the enemy of sun worshippers trying to get a "healthy-looking tan." Now, however, skin cancer is known to be one of those equal opportunity diseases, showing no prejudice toward any skin color. So when you begin looking for a skin care system, get one with sunscreen UV protection and use it no matter what time of year it is.

Facials

Another essential element of good skin care is the facial. While most of us consider having a facial to be somewhat of an extravagance, it should be a part of our overall beauty routine. Facials are deep skin treatments that cleanse, rehydrate, and rejuvenate the skin while reducing skin blemishes, acne, dry skin, and wrinkles. A facial feels good and helps you look your best at any age, but if you start them toward the end of your 20's, you can forestall some of the signs of aging.

A good facial consists of a cleansing procedure, a massage and steam, and a face mask. What this process does is help remove dead skin cells along with pollutants. A massage helps blood circulation, which in turn aids in the removal of toxins and waste from the body. It relaxes facial muscles and helps delay the formation of wrinkles. Steam during a facial helps the skin absorb cream better. It also softens blackheads and whiteheads so that they can be removed easily. Finally, the face mask tones and clarifies the skin, and is effective in treating dry and acne-prone skin.

The type of facial you choose will depend on your skin type.

Basic Facial

In a basic facial the face is first cleansed under steam, then scrub granules are gently massaged over the skin. After removing the scrub, a creamy cleanser is applied using a soft rotating electric brush to further exfoliate the skin. Then the face is gently massaged. Finally, a refreshing toner is applied. This is one of the least expensive facials, and it works well with normal skin. However, this type of cleansing procedure can be used on all skin types for people under 25 years of age. If done regularly, it will reduce many skin problems. (Wouldn't it be nice if someone could do this for us every day?)

Facials for sensitive skin use this same procedure with hypoallergenic products. AHA (alpha hydroxy acid) products derived from fruit acids are used to make the skin appear young and fresh. They are great for cleansing and moisturizing sensitive skin.

Normal Facial

This is the same as a basic facial except the skin is massaged for a longer period of time. Don't get carried away, however. Remember that the tissues of the face are very delicate.

Acne Facial

This facial requires a more complex and expensive treatment. The skin is cleansed, exfoliated, and steamed to clean the pores. These steps are followed by an enzyme or glycolic acid exfoliation and a warm vapor mist, then extensive manual deep pore extractions, electric disencrustation, and a skin-calming, antibacterial mask. This facial should be performed at regular two-week intervals, and may require the assistance of a trained skin care professional.

Collagen Facial

A collagen facial can be used for all skin types. It involves the use of exfoliation, warm vapor, deep pore cleansing, lymphatic drainage massage, and self-healing mineral or paraffin masks over a freeze-dried collagen sheet to ensure the desired hydrating effect. This facial uses the basic facial techniques, but it takes them a step further with collagen sheets to balance moisture. It is very effective against harmful environmental damage.

Bridal Facial

Bridal facials are also known as paraffin facials. Many salons offer them as a part of a woman's bridal day of beauty. A special paraffin mask on the face over layers of gauze (I know it sounds like something out of a mummy film) provides results that are far from hideous as it balances the complexion and makes the face look more radiant.

Special Procedures

As the treatment of skin continues to evolve, women (and men) have more choices to improve their skin's overall appearance through the use of chemical peels and microdermabrasion.

A chemical peel is the removal of the top layer of skin (usually sun damaged) to expose the more evenly textured fresh skin underneath. The idea is to stimulate the production of collagen as an anti-aging factor.

Chemical peels can be performed by licensed estheticians. For deeper skin rejuvenation, however, you would need to visit a dermatologist. It requires a trained medical professional to perform a deep chemical peel.

I'm sure many of us have seen the aftereffects of a chemical peel portrayed on television. The episode of *Sex In The City* when Samantha had one comes to mind. While it was funny to watch on television, there is a far more serious undercurrent at work here. Chemical peels are not to be taken lightly. Before you make an appointment with an esthetician or dermatologist, you should get recommendations from a trusted friend and do your research. This is especially true for women of color. Darker skin tends to suffer from hyper-pigmentation that results in blemishes and marks (this is often a result of squeezing or picking at pimples). Women of color should always seek the advice of a dermatologist who has had experience working with their skin type.

There are many over-the-counter chemical peel kits available for use at home. Before you invest in one, take some time to visit your dermatologist or esthetician for their advice. The chemical solutions in these kits aren't the same concentration as those the professionals use; nevertheless, it's the misuse of the product that can cause damage, so be very careful.

Microdermabrasion is a technique that uses a laser to help repair sun damaged skin and reduce the effects of aging. This procedure should be performed by a trained medical professional—either a dermatologist or a plastic surgeon—since this is a very precise procedure. Again, a note of caution for women of color. This type of technique has the potential to do more damage than good. Schedule a consultation with a doctor to discuss the pros and cons of this procedure for your skin.

Home Facials

If finances are a concern, here are some great do-it-yourself-at-home facials from an article in Redbook Magazine.[†]

"While a dermatologist is trained to treat skin problems, an esthetician is trained to get skin looking and feeling its best," says 45-year-old Esta Kronberg, M.D., who works with an esthetician in her Houston medical office. [Redbook] asked three of these skin pros to share their personal at-home recipes. Whip one up at least once a month for fabulous skin.

[†]Article originally published in Redbook Magazine. Used with permission.

Normal/Oily Skin
Yasmine Djerradine, esthetician and spa owner in New York City

Ingredients:
1 Tablespoon yeast
1 Tablespoon baking soda
1 Teaspoon water

Mix ingredients together and apply (after cleansing) from forehead to collarbone. Allow mask to sit for 15 minutes as the yeast deep cleans and tightens pores and the baking soda evens out blotchiness. (Note: it will not dry or harden.) Rinse with warm water and follow with an oil-free moisturizer.

Normal/Dry Skin:
Andrea Stotsky, esthetician and national trainer for Decleor

Ingredients:
2 Tablespoons honey
1/2 Cup plain yogurt (not low-fat)
1 Teaspoon grapefruit zest
1 Cup iced black tea

Combine first three ingredients and apply mixture to your clean face and neck. Leave mask on for at least 15 minutes. The honey acts like a giant sponge, pulling out impurities and brightening the skin, while the yogurt moisturizes and softens. (The grapefruit scent is energizing.) Splash off with the tea, then massage in your usual day cream.

Sensitive/Irritated Skin:
Regina Viotto, spa director of The Paul Lebreque Salon in New York City

Ingredients:
1 Teaspoon chickpea flour (available in natural health food stores)
1 Teaspoon heavy cream
2 Teaspoons salt water
Pinch of salt

Mix and distribute this creamy concoction all over your clean face. Leave on for ten minutes to let the chickpea flour deep clean stressed skin while the heavy cream balances its pH level (imbalance is what makes sensitive skin red). Rinse with cool water.

MAKEUP

Believe it or not, facial shape and structure play a big role in makeup application. Attractive features should be emphasized, while asymmetrical features should be downplayed. The following are some guidelines for makeup application:

Working With Your Face Shape

Oval Faces

Oval is the most symmetrical face shape, and there is little need for corrective makeup. The eyebrows should flow into a natural arch. If you are unsure of what your natural arch is, leave your arch alone for at least a month and resist the urge to pluck or wax. Your natural arch will become apparent and you can pluck or wax accordingly. Apply blush color in a "C" shape, blending upward toward the eyes.

Oblong and Rectangular Faces

The objective here is to reduce the length of the face. To accomplish this, a darker shade of foundation is applied to the top of the forehead and across the jaw and chin. Eye makeup should make the eyes appear wider and therefore balance the forehead. Blush application should not be higher than the corner of the eyes and should not dip below the nose. The eyebrows should be slightly thick, and your natural arch will further reduce face length.

Round Faces

Round faces are almost equal in width and length. The objective is to play down fullness and emphasize length to achieve an oval look. To accomplish this, apply darker foundation around the sides of the face,

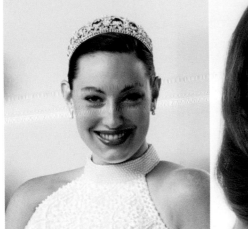
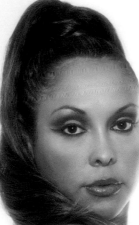
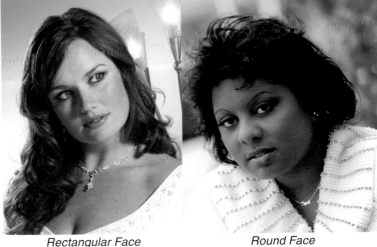

| *Oval Face* | *Oblong Face* | *Rectangular Face* | *Round Face* |

the jawline, and under the cheeks. This will make the forehead look narrow and draw the eye downward, thus achieving an elongated look. Apply blush directly on the cheekbones and blend toward the temples. The eyebrows should be somewhat longer to frame the eyes; this can be achieved through eyebrow maintenance or with the help of a brow pencil.

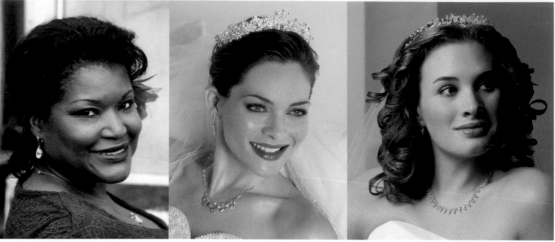

Heart-shaped Face   Square Face   Diamond Face

Heart-shaped Faces

A heart-shaped face is characterized by a wide forehead and narrow chin. The objective is to make the chin and jawline appear wider. Apply a darker shade of foundation to minimize the forehead and use a lighter shade of foundation to widen the jawline. Additionally, you can use white eye shadow around the side of the cheeks to create width. Blush should be applied on the upper cheek. Eyebrows should be somewhat thick (not bushy) and straight (not too straight). They should follow a natural arch, but with a little distance between the brows.

Square Faces

This is the strongest facial shape. It is characterized by a straight forehead and a square jawline. The objective is to soften the edges, which can be done by applying a darker shade of foundation to the temple area, jawline, and sides of the face. Apply blush on the cheeks and blend it toward the jawline to add length to the face. Lipstick has to be applied to create fullness in the lips; this will divert attention from the square jawline. Eyebrows should be rounded in shape to make the face appear softer.

Diamond-shaped Faces

A diamond-shaped face is characterized by a narrow forehead and chin with wide cheek bones. Makeup should be applied to reduce the width of the cheeks and make the face appear more oval in shape. To achieve this, apply a darker shade of foundation to the outer corners of the cheekbones and blend upward toward the eyes. Then apply a lighter shade of foundation to the chin and the forehead, which creates the illusion of width. Eyebrows should be slightly apart from the center, and should flow into the natural arch.

Triangular Faces

This facial shape is characterized by a narrow forehead, a wide jawline, and a wide chin. The goal of makeup application here is to add width to the forehead and length to the face overall. To achieve this look, use a darker foundation around the sides of the face to reduce the width of the jawline. Blush should be applied on the cheekbones and blended toward the jawline to balance the face and create the illusion of an oval-shaped face. Eyebrows should be shaped to create a higher arch on the outer ends.

Eyes and Eyebrows

Eyes are considered the windows of the soul, and like most windows, they need to be dressed up to highlight their shape and beauty. Just as faces and bodies come in many different shapes, the same is true of eyes. Therefore, it is essential to know the shape of your eyes in order to bring out their best.

Wide Set Eyes

Wide Set Eyes seem to be set far apart on the face. You can do several things to make them appear closer together:

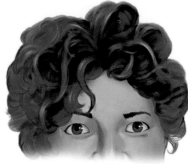

- Use deep colors near the inner corners of the eyes. This will give the illusion of your eyes being closer.

- Use medium colored shadow on the eyelids and creases, and focus color application on the inner corners.

- Use eyeliner to make your eyes pop.

- Use a volume-building mascara.

Close Set Eyes

Close Set Eyes appear closer to the bridge of the nose. In order to open your eyes up, do the direct opposite of the techniques for wide set eyes:

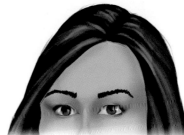

- Apply deep colors to the outer corners of the eyes; this gives the illusion of width.

- Eyeliner applied in a line will make your eyes appear smaller, so if you use eyeliner, smudge it to open up the eyes.

Evenly Spaced Eyes

Evenly Spaced Eyes allow for more options in eye makeup color and application. Special shading techniques are not necessary.

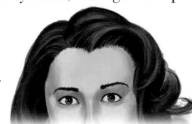

Almond Eyes

Almond Eyes with a slight turn at the corner are considered an ideal shape as well. They also allow for more highlighting color options.

- Use eyeliner on the upper and lower lids.
- Light eye shadow can be used from the lashes to the eyebrow.
- Use a medium shade eye shadow on the eyelids themselves.
- Follow up with a darker shade on the outer part of the eyelid.
- Finish with mascara to make the eyes pop.

Oriental Eyes

Oriental Eyes are similar to almond eyes, except they have a little more lift in the corners. However, the eyelids are recessed, unlike the almond shape where the eyelid crease is clearly defined. Just as you want to make the eyes pop for almond-shaped eyes, you want to do the same thing for oriental eyes in order to draw attention to the eyes and not the fact that the lids are recessed.

- Use dark, smoky eye shadow at the base of the eye.
- Follow up with a similarly colored eyeliner in the same area.

Small Eyes

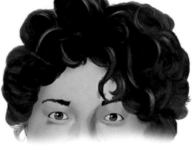

Small Eyes are smaller in comparison to other facial features. The objective here is to open the eyes and make them appear larger to balance the face.

- Use an eyelash curler.
- When using liner, only line the bottom of the eye. If you line the top, you are closing the eye and making it appear even smaller.
- Use light colored eye shadow to create width.
- Use medium colored shadow on the crease of the eye.

Large Eyes

Large Eyes tend to dominate facial features.

- Use deeper shades of eye shadow to make eyes appear smaller.
- Use liner at the base of the eye and blend it to the corner for a more exotic look.

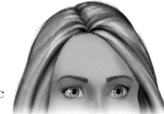

Hooded Eyes

Hooded Eyes are characterized by eyelids that seem nonexistent. Makeup needs to bring the eyes forward with clever shaping and shading techniques.

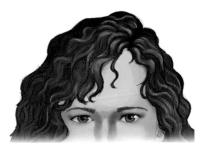

- Use a medium to dark colored shadow on the eye crease.

- Use mascara on the upper lashes but not on the lower lashes. Mascara on the lower lashes draws attention to the nonexistent looking eyelids.

Deep Set Eyes

Deep Set Eyes are recessed and need to pop. To bring them out you can:

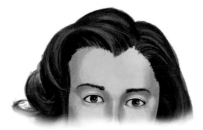

- Choose light colored shadows to enhance the eyes.

- Use deep colors on the brow bone.

Eyebrows

If the eyes are the windows of the soul, then eyebrows serve as their frame. There is an art to the shaping of brows, and it should be based on your natural arch. Estheticians use several techniques to achieve this goal, but only you can decide which one works best for you:

Tweezing is a tried and true method. Hairs are plucked one by one with tweezers. This is a great method because it can be done at home or at a salon. The downside is it can be painful and it doesn't remove all the fine hairs. It usually lasts four to eight weeks, depending upon your regrowth rate.

Threading uses a cotton thread to twist out several or more hairs at a time, and it is reported to be less irritating. The downside is it doesn't remove the hair from the root. It also lasts between four and eight weeks.

Permanent Hair Removal should be performed by a skin care professional or dermatologist. This method uses a laser to kill hair at the root. The upside is it removes hair permanently. The downside is you must find a skilled professional to avoid injury and burning.

Waxing is the most common method for eyebrows. A honey-based wax is applied to the brow, covered with fabric, and removed quickly to pull the hairs. The upside is it removes all hair, including the fine and coarse hairs. It usually lasts from four to eight weeks. You must be careful to go to a trusted salon so the shape (arch) of your brow is maintained.

Lip Shapes

The one essential all women carry with them is a tube of lipstick. If I put nothing else on my face, I always have a little blush and lipstick on—otherwise I feel unfinished. And I'm not alone. Most women consider lipstick a priority. However, while we love lipstick, there is an art to applying it for maximum effect. Once again it is about shape; the shape of your lips will determine how you should and shouldn't apply lip color.

Full Lips

Full Lips are characterized by a generous upper and lower lip. In order to make them appear less full, use neutral to dark tones with a matte look. Glossy lipsticks will make the lips appear larger. Also, when lining lips, do so on the inside of the lip line and make sure the lip liner isn't too dark. It should be in the same shade family as the lipstick.

Thin Lips

Thin Lips are long and almost straight in appearance. To give them shape and depth, line the outer part of the lip with a light to medium-light shade. When choosing lip color, choose glossy lipsticks. This will make the lips appear larger. Stay away from matte lipstick shades. They make lips appear even smaller and almost cartoonish.

Down-turned Lips

Down-turned Lips have an unhappy bend to them. To raise their spirits, use a little concealer or foundation in the corner of the lips; then use a lip liner (or pencil) to draw a happy smile.

Unbalanced Lips

Unbalanced Lips occur when one lip is smaller or larger than the other. To balance them, match one with the other. In other words, if your top lip is more prominent, use a lip liner on the inside of the lip line to make the bottom one balance—and vice versa.

Balanced Lips

Balanced Lips are the perfect shape. You can choose to enhance them however you want using lipstick with a matte or high gloss finish.

Vague Lips

Vague Lips are not readily visible. Therefore, you can draw the shape with a lip pencil and fill it in with lip color.

Makeup for the Plus-size Bride

You may be wondering if you should be doing anything different with your makeup as a plus-size bride. There are a few techniques you can try, but for the most part you can do your makeup like anyone else. The only real differences in plus-size women's faces is that they are fuller and may have large cheeks or double chins. These differences don't change their beauty, but if your intention is to make your face look slimmer, there are a few tricks that you or your makeup artist can use.

You may have heard the words "contouring" and "highlighting" before. These techniques use darker or lighter makeup in certain areas to play up or minimize features.

Contouring is the process of adding darker color to certain areas of your face to make them recede and look thinner or less prominent. Contouring can be done with a powder or cream. Many makeup artists choose a beige- or brown-toned blush or shadow. "Tropical" shadow by Paula Dorf is great, but will not work on very dark skin. MAC makes some excellent blushes, such as "Reed," that darker women can use.

Some makeup artists use a foundation stick instead of a powder to contour. In this case, they will choose a foundation two to three shades darker than your skin. The skill with either of these products is knowing how and where to apply them. This needs to be done with caution, or you will end up looking like you have brown smudges or stripes on your face.

The time to contour is after you have applied your foundation and concealer. Some makeup artists also apply face powder first, but that's up to you. The first and most obvious place to contour is your cheeks. Suck in your cheeks to find your cheekbones. Use a contour brush or angled blush brush and apply a line of color to the hollowed area of your cheekbone and slightly below. If you did this correctly you should be able to see right away the slimming effect it has on your face.

Chances are this will look very dramatic initially. Now take a clean sponge and softly blend the color down in short rounded strokes. Then take a clean blush brush and rub it over the contoured area in gentle circles, blending the color so it doesn't have a hard line. Apply a translucent face powder to further soften the look. Finally, add a soft pink- or peach-toned blush to the apples of your cheeks only. If you have very large cheeks, do not use a blush with shimmer as it will make the cheeks look larger.

If you feel like you did a good job on your cheeks, you can experiment with other areas of your face—but it is not quite as easy. Generally, the other areas you might want to contour are the jawline and directly under your chin (to minimize a double chin). If applied too heavily, this will look like you have stripes of dirt on your neck. Use a light touch.

Now that you have finished contouring, you can start highlighting. Highlighting is the technique of adding a light color or shimmer to bring an area of the face forward and accentuate it. Highlighting, like contouring, needs to be done carefully and subtly. There are a few great products you can use for highlighting. Prescriptives Sheen Cream in "Beam" looks fantastic on the temples. It is a subtle golden shade, and makes you look brighter, more awake, and shimmery. Benefit also makes two really nice highlighters: a pink tone called "Moonbeam," and a gold tone called "Highbeam."

For highlighting other areas of your face, it's best to use a foundation color two to three shades lighter than your foundation color. The best place to apply this light foundation color is to the area of your cheeks below the area where you contoured. Highlighting here will bring this area of your face forward and will further recess the contoured area, making your cheekbones look even more defined. Again, follow the same steps of blending with a sponge, making circles with a clean blush brush, and then applying more face powder.

Other than these contouring and highlighting steps, you can apply your makeup the same way anyone else would.

A Professional's View of Makeup

Creating the perfect look for your face is as important as it is with your hair. As a full-figured woman, I am sure you have been told "what a pretty face" you have. Now it's time to accentuate the positive, and for that we turn to an expert.

As an experienced professional makeup artist, Lisa Alpern is one of the most highly sought professionals in her field. Located in New York City, Lisa works with a few select hairstylists for weddings so that she can provide the complete package to brides. These stylists all work for top New York City salons.

Professionally known as Lisafashionista, in addition to weddings, Lisa does editorial and commercial print work. She works with musicians (producing album covers, among other things), fashion designers (for look books and promotional materials), and actors and actresses (headshots). She also teaches makeup lessons to individuals and aspiring makeup artists.

Lisa has started her own online magazine for plus-size women called Beauty Plus Power (www.beautypluspower.com). The magazine focuses on many different aspects of life (relationships, health, self-esteem, and fashion) as they relate to plus-size women. The site is working toward building the largest online shopping guide available for plus-size women in categories ranging from costumes, to lingerie, to workout wear, and much more. Lisa is a plus-size woman herself and believes that size has very little to do with success or happiness.

Moreover, as a plus-size woman she has firsthand knowledge of how to create the perfect makeup look for full-figured women, and she has been kind enough to share it with us on her web site.

Makeup is a great way to accentuate your natural beauty. It can transform your look from everyday to glamorous, much like your wedding gown.

Who Will Do Your Makeup?

Several months in advance, consider whether you want to do your own makeup. This may not be an easy decision to make. You have probably already discovered that weddings can be quite expensive. Hiring a makeup artist would be one more expense. On a positive note, your makeup will most assuredly cost less than the flowers, the food, or the location! Here are some questions to help you decide.

Do you:

- Have good skin?

- Wear makeup everyday?

- Get complimented frequently on your makeup?

- Own a good selection of makeup products?

- Feel comfortable applying dramatic makeup?

- Dislike having someone else touch your face?

- Have trouble trusting others to do your makeup?

If you answered "yes" to most of these questions, you may be capable of doing your own makeup for your wedding. This is a good choice for people who like being in control, but it requires skill, patience, and confidence. It is not advisable to make this choice if you never wear makeup or own very little makeup. You may not have sufficient experience (or resources) to create the look you want.

Ask yourself if you:

- Have the budget to hire a makeup artist (anywhere from $75–$500).

- Feel it would be stressful to do your own makeup.

- Have acne or uneven skin tone.

- Sweat a lot.

- Have very dry or very oily skin.

- Want to be pampered on your wedding day.

If you answered "yes" to most of these questions, consider hiring a professional. Makeup artists are aware of how different products will photograph, and they can prevent you from looking shiny or ghostly pale in your pictures. If you have very dry or oily skin, there are techniques a makeup artist can use to minimize these problems. It is also very easy for makeup artists to cover acne or discoloration, as they have a lot of experience in blending and evening skin tone. Trials beforehand will let you know what to expect so there will be no surprises.

Now that you have considered the benefits of each of these options, you can make an informed decision. The next two sections will cover what to expect if you are doing your own makeup, and what to expect if you are hiring a makeup artist. Even if you have already made your choice, it could be beneficial to read more about each option.

Doing Your Own Makeup

Before we start, there are some basics you must decide. First, do you know what you want to look like on your wedding day? Have you always envisioned yourself as a dramatic bride with glamorous makeup, or did you picture yourself looking very natural? If you already have an idea, that's great! But don't panic if you aren't sure. Look through the bridal and fashion magazines around your house and rip out some pictures you like. Also, look at makeup books for ideas, such as Kevyn Aucoin's *Making Faces*, or Reggie Wells' *Face Painting*.

Once you have selected a picture for inspiration, consider whether you have the necessary products to complete your look. Examine your makeup collection. Some of your products may need to be replaced. Mascara should be changed every three months; older mascaras will solidify, causing clumpy, dry looking lashes. Liquid foundations last about a year before they start to separate. Lipsticks tend to dry out in approximately two years and may make your lips look waxy.

Now take a look at your brush collection. Do you have professional quality brushes from a department store, or are your brushes from a drug store or a free gift you received when you purchased some other product? Quality brushes make a huge difference in makeup application. Your products will spread more evenly and look truer to color. Some of the companies that sell quality brushes are MAC, Bobbi Brown, Shu Uemera, Paula Dorf, Estée Lauder, Sephora, Iman, Lancôme, Maybelline, Max Factor, Revlon, and Smashbox. Check one of these lines for a prepackaged brush set, or consider the following individual brushes:

- Large Powder Brush: the bigger the better.

- Blush Brush: this will normally look like a smaller version of a powder brush.

- Eyebrow Brush: look for an angled brush with very tight, short bristles.

- Three Shadow Brushes: a fluff brush for lids, a chiseled fluff for contouring, and a small rounded brush for doing stronger contouring or highlighting.

- Straight Liner Brush: if you like to put powder eyeliner on, this is the best brush to use.

- Lip Brush: find a retractable lip brush with a top so you can put it in your touch-up kit.

- Cheek Contour brush (optional): this brush often looks like a giant angled shadow brush. It is used to define cheekbones and bring out your features.

Brushes are just the beginning. You will also need to determine which products are necessary for you. Below is a list of products you might use. Those in *italics* are products the average person may not have or know how to use. It might be worth experimenting with them if you are skilled at doing your makeup, but you can still do a beautiful job without these extra products. The products are listed in the order they should be applied (keep in mind you will select from some of these products—don't try to use them all at the same time). For more information about these products, consult the Makeup Appendix on page 131.

For Your Face

Eye cream
Moisturizer
Primer
Concealer
Foundation
Blush
Contour color
Highlighter
Powder
Fixative

For Your Eyes

Base shadow
Contour shadow
Highlight shadow
Eyelash curler
Eyeliner
Mascara or Clear mascara
Individual false eyelashes
Lash glue
Tweezers
Eyebrow pencil or wax
Brow gel

For Your Lips

Lip primer
Lip pencil liner
Lipstick
Lip sealant
Lip gloss

You may be wondering where to purchase these products. If you feel that you are capable of picking things out without a sales assistant, try Sephora. This makeup store is found in malls around the country. It carries so many different lines of makeup that you will probably be able to find whatever you need.

If you are not comfortable picking out the shades you want, go to your local higher-end department store, like Saks or Bloomingdale's. Choose a makeup counter that you trust and have an associate pick out products with you. MAC, Benefit, Trish McEvoy, Lancôme, Smashbox, Estée Lauder, Prescriptives, Clinique, Iman, Fashion Fair, and Bobbi Brown all offer excellent products for bridal makeup.

Now that you have bought all the right products, it's time to try them out. Set aside at least an hour to practice. Find a place with good natural light and space to lay out everything you need. Beware of fluorescent light because it will emphasize all your flaws and distort the colors.

Practice when you are wearing no makeup at all, ideally right after you shower, so you are starting with a clean face. Start by moisturizing your skin, paying extra attention to dry spots. No matter what your skin type is, moisturizers are very beneficial. A well-moisturized face will not need to produce as much oil to keep the skin hydrated, so you will not get as shiny. In addition, moisturizers provide a smooth surface on which to apply your makeup. Wait at least five minutes to start your makeup after you have applied your moisturizer

Here are a few tips to guide you when applying your makeup:

- A good quality sponge can make your foundation spread more smoothly. You can buy sponges inexpensively by the dozen from a makeup supply store called Alcone (www.alconeco.com). These sponges are far superior to those available in drug stores.

- There are makeup artists who say you should use a lighter colored concealer than your foundation. This can make you look like a raccoon. Try to match your concealer to your foundation. If you are using a cream or stick foundation, you may not even need a separate concealer.

- Most people know that curling your eyelashes before you put on mascara will amplify them. Curling your eyelashes a second time after you put mascara on will make them look even longer. You may have heard that curling mascara-coated lashes can break them. Unless you are wearing two tons of hardened mascara, this won't happen. Just be gentle and don't pull on your lashes.

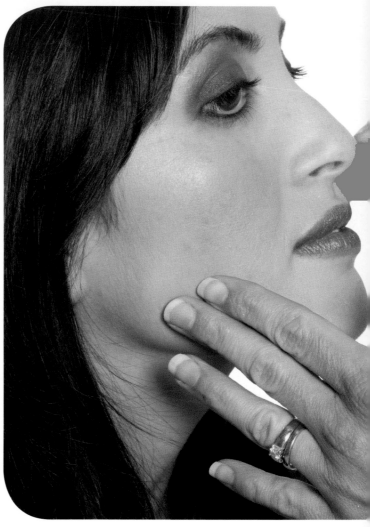

- When applying lip liner, make sure to fill in your whole lip with the liner. If you just line the outside, that's all that will be left when your lipstick wears off.

- Eye shadow color choices for brides are very basic. Use soft colors on your lids like beige, lilac, or baby pink. For your contour color, choose a darker shade, such as an eggplant or brown. For your highlighter, stick to a pale shimmery white or peach.

When you have finished doing the trial run on your makeup, take a good look in the mirror. Are you happy with the result? Look at it from close up and far away, in indoor and outdoor light. Have someone take pictures so you can see how it looks on film. Pictures can also give you a guide to use when doing your makeup again on your wedding day.

What if you hate the way you did your makeup? Will practice make perfect? Try doing it again a few more times to see if there is any improvement. If you think it's a failure, now is the time to consider hiring a makeup artist. This may be what you were trying to avoid, but you want to look your best on your wedding day. The next section will give you an idea of where to begin your search if you choose to hire someone.

Hiring a Makeup Artist

You may already have a makeup artist in mind for your wedding, whether it is a friend of a friend, or your favorite salesgirl at the department store makeup counter. If you don't already have an idea, here are some suggestions for finding one.

The first thing to do when searching for a makeup artist is to ask around. If you have friends who had beautiful makeup at their weddings, ask them who did it. If you are the first of your friends to get married or no one has a recommendation, there are great online communities for brides, such as www.theknot.com. Online communities often have specific sections where makeup artists can pay to advertise. There are also public forums where people can leave feedback about a bridal makeup artist. Or you can do a web search for makeup artists in your area. There are tons of makeup artists who have their own websites. Many of these makeup artists work in TV, film, or print, but do weddings on the side. So don't rule them out if you like their work.

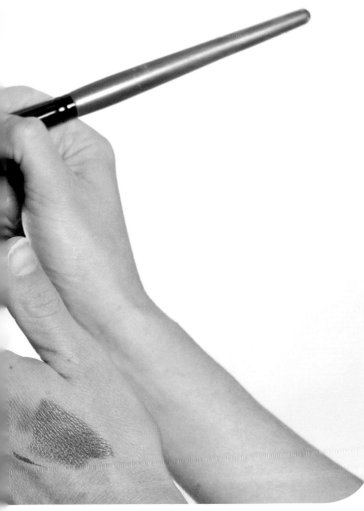

Regardless of where you heard about a makeup artist, or how highly they come recommended, there are many questions to ask. First, make sure they have your wedding date available! Next find out how much they charge for trials. Trial prices vary by city and by individual artist. You can expect to hear anything from $25.00 to $100.00. Artists often have high trial fees because of the time and energy it takes to do a bridal consultation. It would be unusual to find someone who offers a free trial, because most makeup artists cannot afford to offer their services for free.

Ask for a price quote for the wedding prior to the trial. Makeup artists generally charge one price for brides, and a less expensive price for wedding party members (sometimes half of what they charge the bride). Some makeup artists may have additional fees. They may charge for transportation or gas money. They may also charge an extra fee for early morning hours. Keep in mind that bridal makeup can be very expensive. However, if the price sounds unusually high to you, call other makeup artists in your area and compare. Once you find an affordable makeup artist that you like, arrange a trial right away.

When you go to a trial, the makeup artist should have some questions for you. They will probably ask if you brought pictures of your desired look. If you didn't bring any, they should ask questions about what you want to look like. They should also ask how you normally wear your makeup so they can get an idea of your preferences. They may ask about the dress, the veil, the time of year, the time of day, and the location. These are all questions that can give them an idea of what is appropriate for you. Additionally, they should ask you if you have any allergies to makeup products. If they don't ask, and you do in fact have allergies, please make sure to mention it to them!

At the trial, take a look at the makeup artist's kit. Makeup artists are rarely if ever completely brand loyal. You will probably see a variety of high and low end products, but don't expect the whole kit to look like a makeup counter. Check to see if their products look clean and observe their methods when applying makeup. Are they using sanitary practices, such as using disposable mascara wands and spraying lipsticks with alcohol before applying? Did they wash their hands before they started, or clean them with a baby wipe or hand sanitizer? Don't be afraid to ask questions about their kit sanitation.

It is also important to consider the personality of the makeup artist. Are they nice, warm, and personable? Are they critical? Do they seem to be rushing you? On your wedding day, you will likely be stressed and a little nervous. You want to feel at ease with your makeup artist. They should treat you with kindness and respect, and be focused on doing a great job.

Take note of how long it takes them to apply your makeup. Ask if this is how long it will take on your wedding day. If they take an hour and a half at your trial, but tell you it will take 20 minutes on your wedding day, be suspicious. Keep in mind that the trial generally takes a little longer than your wedding day makeup because they will be asking questions and trying things out. It is fairly standard to leave about an hour for the bride, although there are many artists who do brides in less time. But why try to rush them? This is your special day and you want to look your best. As for your bridesmaids, they will most likely quote you a time of between 20–45 minutes each.

Once your makeup is done, you have to decide if you like it. Check it in natural light if possible since makeup looks a lot different in fluorescent light. If you really hate it or don't like the makeup artist, pay the artist and go home. If it's a disaster now, it will be a disaster at your wedding. If you are unsure, or there are certain aspects you like and certain you don't, don't be afraid to ask for changes. This is what the trial is for! They may not have a clear sense of what you are looking for, and you can help explain it to them. Of course, you may be thrilled by the makeup and want to hire the makeup artist on the spot.

Once you are ready to hire an artist, there are important things to discuss with him or her. One thing you may want to talk about is discounts. Most makeup artists are not going to offer a discount on the bride, but it's very possible that if you bring them a big wedding party, say four or five bridesmaids, they may be willing to give you a little price break. The bigger the wedding party, the better the chance that you will get a discount. Always make sure you're nice and not pushy when you ask—but don't be afraid to try. The worst thing the artist can say is no!

Some makeup artists will have a standard contract for you to sign. Others don't use a contract at all. *YOU WANT A CONTRACT.* This document protects you and your makeup artist. Following are some topics that should be covered in the contract:

- How much of a deposit is required to validate the contract? It's always best to have money-related matters in writing. Make sure you give the deposit amount in the form of a check. For trials, however, you can pay in cash.

- Who does the deposit cover? If you are paying the total cost for your mother, sister, and aunt, but not for your friend, you want to make sure it says that in the contract. If you put a deposit in the contract for a friend and that friend later cancels, you will be the one held financially responsible.

- Are deposits refundable? The general answer to this is no, but read below about cancellations and refunds.

- What services are being guaranteed in the contract? Make sure that the contract specifies who is getting what service (especially important if you hire a makeup artist who is also doing hair).

- How many people are being covered in the contract? As with the deposit, the contract should list the people who will be using the services of your makeup artist. Be sure to only list the names of people whose services you will be guaranteeing financially.

- Who will be performing the services? Make sure it says that your makeup artist is responsible for makeup application on your wedding day. Then on the day of the wedding if a stranger shows up and says your makeup artist hired her to do your makeup, you will not be obligated to pay.

- What money needs to be paid or refunded in the event of a cancellation? This will protect both of you. Your artist may have certain rules, such as if you cancel with less than a 30-day notice, you have to pay 50% of the total cost. If your artist cancels on you, make sure you can get your deposit back. Read through this section of the contract carefully so that you understand your rights. Generally, if you cancel you will not get your deposit back. If they cancel, you should get all the money back.

- What happens if your artist arrives late? Make sure the contract states that if the artist is more than a certain amount of time late (e.g., 30 minutes), there is a specified discount on services.

- What happens if you arrive late? This is to protect the artist more than you, but you should respect them enough to agree to this. You can't really expect them to finish their services at the time you planned if you show up an hour late.

- What happens if the artist is late finishing your services? This circumstance should also be covered by a discount clause. However, there might be extenuating circumstances, so make sure those are written in as well.

Note that there are exceptions to any situation that can be written into the contract. If one of you is late because you overslept, that's obviously someone's fault. But if one of you is late because there was a four-foot snowstorm, then neither of you is to blame. So you can add something about weather, natural disasters, road closures, health issues, and other factors if you want.

The final thing you need to do is go over all the preparation plans for your wedding day with your makeup artist. The more information you give the professional the better. Here are some things he or she will need to know:

- Contact phone numbers for you prior to the event.

- Contact phone numbers for the day of the event.

- Emergency contact numbers for the day of the event.

- Contact numbers for your hairstylist (to coordinate schedule planning if necessary).

- The time when the ceremony starts.

- The time when the bridal party needs to be ready.

- The time when the pictures start.

- Where you are getting ready for the wedding, and directions to that location.

- What time you want the artist to arrive.

Here is an easy way to calculate preparation time: typically, the bride will need one hour for her make-up, and her bridesmaids will need between twenty and forty-five minutes each. Tell your makeup artist that you would also like to leave twenty or thirty minutes extra as a time cushion. Finally, makeup artists should never do the bride last, because if things are running late, the bride is not the person whose makeup should be rushed!

Your Touch-up Kit

Whether you are doing your own makeup or hiring a professional, you will need to prepare a touch-up kit. This way you can fix your makeup after the ceremony or during the reception. With just a few products by your side, you can look fabulous all night long. Here are the essentials:

Powder

If you do your own makeup: Even if you normally use a loose powder, purchase a pressed powder to put in your touch-up kit. It's less messy and very portable.

If you hire a makeup artist: The artist may use loose or pressed powder. If he uses pressed powder during your trial, ask for the brand and consider purchasing it yourself. If he uses loose powder, he will most likely be using a powder puff to apply it. Ask if he can fill the puff with more powder and then put it in a resealable bag for you.

Lipstick

If you do your own makeup: Bring your lipstick with you.

If you hire a makeup artist: If your artist uses a lipstick color you love, ask what it is during the trial and consider purchasing it. If he mixes a custom color for you, ask for a little sample in a plastic container to put in your touch-up kit. The artist may even have a disposable lip brush to give you. If not, buy a re-tractable lip brush so you can put it in your touch-up kit without making a mess.

Cotton Swabs

If you cry during the ceremony, you may end up smudging your makeup. Use waterproof products to avoid this as much as possible. Even if you aren't a crier, your makeup may run a little bit. Whatever the reason, it's just a good idea to have a couple of cotton swabs on hand to wipe away anything that might drop or smudge.

Mirror

This one is obvious. How can you check your makeup if you don't have a mirror with you? Powder, lip-stick, Q-tips, and a mirror are really the only essentials a bride can't live without in her touch-up kit. Items like nail polish, lip gloss, eye shadow and concealer are optional. It all depends on how much touching up you want to do. No amount is too little or too much, but don't forget to enjoy yourself. You don't want to run off every five seconds during your reception to check your face.

Now the question is—where to put your kit? You obviously aren't going to be strutting down the aisle with a purse! If you only want to touch up between the ceremony and the reception, you can keep a little kit in your bridal prep room (if your location has one). If not, consider getting a chic white purse and filling it with the products you need. Then have your maid of honor make sure that it gets placed on your table at the reception so you have it available.

If you want to know more about makeup products, take a look at the Makeup Appendix on page 131.

MANICURES AND PEDICURES

This touch feels like a major indulgence. What could be better than letting someone make your hands and feet feel beautiful. If you are getting married in the evening, you might consider having your nails (and the wedding party's nails) done the day of the wedding. Many nail salons provide in-home service for just such occasions. However, if your wedding is taking place in the morning or early afternoon, schedule everyone's nails for the day before.

Choosing the color of your nail polish is a way to state your personal style as it relates to the season. If your wedding is in the fall, perhaps you would choose a vibrant color that reflects the season's change. Flesh tone shades have also been gaining in popularity. Years ago, women of color were often subjected to the too-light champagnes and beiges worn by their white counterparts. Today, nail polish manufacturers are jumping on the bandwagon of actual flesh tones in droves. In fact, the once classic white French manicure has been altered to match darker skin tones.

Then, of course, for the more daring of us, there is airbrushing designs on our nails. If you don't have naturally long nails and want to have tips put on for your wedding day, make sure you begin the practice well before the wedding. Having long nails when you're not used to them takes some practice, so give yourself time to become accustomed to them.

Pedicures seem to be of particular importance if your wedding is in the summer months and you will be wearing an open-toe shoe. Although it's the most obvious reason for a pedicure, a more important reason to have one is to counteract the standing, walking, and dancing you are going to put your feet through, regardless of the time of year. Your feet deserve to be pampered.

HAIR REMOVAL

Of all the things women do to pamper themselves, waxing is the least soothing. But it is a necessary evil.

Lip and Chin

Wouldn't it be great if the hair on our heads grew as fast as it does on our faces? It's a nice thought, but it won't happen. At one time or another, we've all stood in front of the mirror with a pair of tweezers for a "clean up." In order to avoid this for your wedding, it has been suggested that you wax as close to the date as possible. This doesn't present a problem for most women. If you have a tendency to be red for a day or two afterwards, however, make your appointment accordingly to avoid the Botox look.

Eyebrows

Out of all the facial waxing services, the eyebrows are the most important area. The eyebrows serve to frame your lovely eyes and face, so you need to choose the right technician to shape your brow to best fit your face. No "Model T" assembly line eyebrows. It may cost you a bit more, but it's worth it. (The problem with redness after a treatment especially applies to eyebrows.)

Legs

For many of us, a bikini wax (aka leg waxing) is the grooming equivalent of a root canal. Done approximately every two to three weeks, depending on the time of year, it is not only a painful proposition, it's an expensive one. To avoid the lobster look, make your appointment anywhere from three to five days before the wedding.

A note about Brazilian Bikini Wax. It's very popular and very intimate—think of it as leg waxing that encroaches on areas most of us don't expose to anyone but our husbands. You can choose to go the South American way with a "landing strip," or you can dare to go bare. However, use caution when choosing a professional or salon; this is a very intimate process and you want to ask friends for recommendations.

BEING AT YOUR PERSONAL BEST

We've covered all the trappings that surround the wedding day itself, but before we embark on planning your actual wedding, it's time to talk about taking care of yourself. With the busy lives we lead, that can be a tall order. We always seem to put our needs on the back burner. Getting married and planning a wedding is a very wonderful—yet very stressful—time, so we need to find the time to take care of ourselves physically and emotionally.

Whether you are a size 14, 16, 20, or more, the important thing is to feel good—not only for your wedding, but all the time. Being health conscious has absolutely nothing to do with our weight or dress size. It is important for us to maintain a healthy balance in order to keep up with the demands in our lives. Most of us wear many hats over the course of a day, so it's easy to fall into bad eating, exercising, and sleeping patterns in the interest of saving time. However, if we don't take action with our health, time won't be on our side.

Diet and Exercise

We have all seen the food pyramid listing the major food groups with its recommended number of servings for each category. It provides a good blueprint for what we need to maintain our health. Nonetheless, it is only a guideline. Only you and your doctor know what's best, and together you can design a health plan to fit your life. Remember, there is no quick fix to being healthy or getting in shape. In other words, you can't lose 60 pounds two months before your wedding—it's unrealistic! The only thing you're guaranteed is disappointment, so why put yourself through it?

A few years ago I worked with a plus-size bride who decided she wanted to lose 75 pounds before her wedding, which completely puzzled me since her fiancé loved and accepted her regardless of the scale or her dress size. According to her, though, she felt she would feel better and be more comfortable if she lost weight.

I couldn't argue with her, but I suggested she set a more reasonable goal. Seventy-five pounds in four months was too much, and could easily have resulted in health problems if not handled properly. So she started eating a healthier, balanced diet with the help of her doctor and a nutritionist, and in the four months before the wedding, she lost a healthy 25 pounds. She looked radiant as she walked down the aisle.

Once again, your comfort is key. The trick is, you can't allow yourself to become obsessed with the scale or the tape measure. You will drive yourself crazy. Instead, as you eat a healthy diet, focus on the extra room you have in the waist of your jeans, or how your favorite blouse fits a bit more smoothly. Stay positive and surround yourself with positive people.

Once you get the green light from your doctor to begin an exercise program, start off slowly. Take it a step at a time and don't set yourself up for failure with unrealistic exercise goals. If you're shy, begin a program at home. Take walks in the morning around your neighborhood. If you prefer a group setting, join a local gym or form your own neighborhood walking/jogging group.

It is essential to feel a sense of belonging when you begin a diet and exercise program. If you want that extra encouragement, try a program like Curves. That's exactly what they focus on. According to CEO and Founder of Curves, Gary Heavin, "Women of all sizes are welcome at Curves. It is important that even full-figured women keep their body fat percentage at healthy levels, strengthen muscles, and stretch for joint health. I don't blame many of them for giving up on weight control due to the defects in the conventional weight loss methods. There is hope. There is help. Curves is a fresh approach that will empower them to successfully control their weight."

That's what it's all about! Empowering yourself with the tools that will add to your happiness. I didn't say make you happy; I said add to your existing happiness. After all, you're marrying the man of your dreams.

Massage Therapy

Taking care of your body isn't all about working up a sweat. Women need to take time to pamper their muscles after a workout through the art of massage.

Getting a massage was once considered something only celebrities or the very rich could afford. However, there has been a boom in spa services in recent years, with more hair and nail salons providing massage therapy. On the other hand, just because a salon offers massages doesn't mean you are getting a "massage therapist"; there is a difference between a massage therapist and a masseuse.

Brenda Mabry, a licensed massage therapist in Virginia Beach, Virginia, explains the difference. "A masseuse is a noncertified body worker. The experience these individuals have had varies from on-the-job training to some formal training, but they have not passed their national certification boards. They can give a relaxing, general massage that is normally done at a spa." Certified Massage Therapists (CMTs) are nationally certified by the National Certification Board for Therapeutic Massage and Bodywork (NCB) to practice the techniques of massage. They're trained in varying techniques for a specific number of hours, which differs from state to state. According to the NCB, a CMT must have completed at least 125 hours of anatomy and physiology, 200 hours of massage and/or bodywork theory and application, 40 hours of pathology, 10 hours of business and ethics, and at least 125 hours of related course work.

Massage therapists are not doctors, but they keep client files—complete with a full medical history, physician's referral, and treatment plans. A good massage therapist knows a medical massage isn't a substitute for seeing a doctor, and will refer all serious medical problems—such as high blood pressure, broken bones, the common cold, etc.—to a physician. Any and all medical problems are addressed at each visit. Massage does aid in overall beneficial health, but as with anything else, the result varies from person to person. The most common benefits of massage are:

- Reduces stress.

- Reduces tension which can cause other medical problems such as headaches, stomach problems, etc.

- Improves recovery from the delivery of a baby, from injuries, and post-surgery.

- Improves circulation.

- Improves sleeping habits.

- Improves flexibility.

So how do you find a good massage therapist? Ask questions like:

- How long have you been a therapist?

- How long have you worked in your present location?

- What types of techniques do you know?

- What hours do you work?

- How long is a regular session and what is the cost?

- What is your appointment cancellation policy?

- Do you take walk-ins or appointments only? (This is where you can tell the difference between a therapist and a body worker. A therapist will normally do appointments only. If they get offended, move on. They aren't for you.)

Sometimes you will find the right therapist the first time around, and other times it may take several different therapists before you find the right one. If you feel uncomfortable, discuss your concerns with them to determine whether they can be resolved, or simply change therapists.

The average therapist knows three to six different massage techniques. The most common are: Swedish massage, Rolfing, sport massage, chair massage, shiatsu, stone massage, and reflexology. These techniques can be used in a variety of soothing ways, as described by Carol A. Canton, a Holistic Therapist in Manorville, New York:

Holistic Massage (reflexology technique)

While medical massage promotes physical health, there are also massage therapists who concentrate on the whole person—with a particular focus on the soul or spirit. Carol Canton specializes in techniques to promote positive energy using all natural essential oils, candles, and aromatic extracts to release negativity and stress.

Healing Stones Massage (stone massage technique)

Another massage option to consider is that of a healing stones massage. The technique is used during a full body massage. Hot stones are immersed in essential oils and placed on areas of discomfort as a point of contact to promote healing. According to Carol Canton, it's beneficial on three levels:

- Physical: It facilitates therapeutic action or benefit to various functions at the physical level.

- Emotional: It facilitates beneficial therapeutic action on the emotional level by providing nurturing, a gentle emotional release.

- Spiritual: It helps return the recipient to his or her original simplicity. It helps the recipient regain equilibrium, a connection to the sweetness of life, and his or her own true nature.

Healing Reflex Massage (reflexology technique)

Aromatic extracts are placed on areas of discomfort with a penetrating therapeutic modality while reflex points in the hands and feet that correlate to the areas of discomfort are stimulated to promote healing. The reflex points are stimulated by stones or pressure, by choice of the therapist. The aromatic extracts may be blended with oil.

Regular deep work on the feet has the ability to reach deeply hidden blockages and set them free in a way you will find amazing. This is not directly treating a disease, but it offers a better flow of energy that will by itself greatly enhance the healing process, whatever other treatment you choose.

Swedish Massage

Long, smooth strokes, incorporating essential oils—very relaxing.

Oriental (Amma) Massage

An ancient form of massage that focuses on balance and movement of energy within the body. It removes blockages, restoring optimum health. Amma is performed with clothes/gown on.

Medical Massage

This is a natural and noninvasive approach to health care. It seeks to support the body's own natural healing capacities. Helpful for arthritis, sciatica, muscle spasms, headache, chronic low back pain, neck and shoulder pain, nasal congestion, and carpal tunnel.

Seated Massage

Designed specifically for upper body, neck, and head. Stone therapy may be incorporated into this treatment.

Therapeutic Stone Massage

Promotes physical and spiritual balancing with the use of volcanic stones, relaxing the body into its deepest level.

Stone/Sole Connection Reflexology

An ancient art of healing with hot/cold stone therapy that promotes physical and spiritual balancing by mapping the body through the feet.

Universal Massage

A customized massage that may include essential oils, hot/cold stones, moist heat, and a vibratory endermatic system. Song pods are used for an overall feeling of peacefulness and relaxation. A heavenly experience!

Queen Esther for Brides (combination of techniques)

This series of spa treatments starts six months to a year before the wedding. (In the Bible, Queen Esther spent six months receiving "oil of Myrrh" treatments and six months with "sweet odours" for purification as she prepared to become the queen of King Ahasuerus [Esther 2:12].)

Queen Esther's royal bath ritual is specifically for the bride-to-be. The treatment begins with a sea salt scrub infused with aromatic oils to be followed by a bath in mineral salts and essential aromatic oils. The last part of the Queen Esther treatment is an aromatherapy full body massage.

Some Queen Esther programs include a "bridal party day" before the spa experience begins where the entire bridal party can indulge in the creative benefits of a massage experience.

Some therapists prefer to use energy techniques as a part of their massage therapy treatment. Reiki and healing touch massage techniques are two types of energy work that are often used alone, or along with the hands-on techniques.

Choosing the right technique differs from person to person. However, if you have "naked" issues, you may want to consider energy work, a chair massage, or reflexology. Also, be sure to consult your doctor before scheduling a massage. He or she may recommend an appropriate technique, normally energy work or a light technique such as Swedish massage (many therapists who are influenced by Hinduism or Buddhism use these light massage techniques).

What to Expect During a Session

The average appointment session will vary based on the type and level of treatment you have. The average session runs from 40–50 minutes, including the pre-interview, review of last visit, and what your needs are at the present time.

At the beginning of each appointment, some of the standard questions are:

1. How was your last treatment?

2. Any problems since the last treatment?

3. Any concerns today?

4. Any changes in your medications?

5. Was there anything you did or didn't like about the last treatment that I should know?

Upon completion of your massage, you will receive follow-up instructions and schedule a follow-up appointment.

Brenda Mabry further states, "A massage therapist lives by the golden rule, DO NO HARM. Some techniques can cause pain but do no harm. Remember to keep the lines of communication open so that if and when pain occurs during a treatment, the adjustment can be made so that you stay within your pain tolerance.

"Knowing and accepting your own body and its faults is the first step in going to a massage therapist. Learning and dealing with what can and cannot be changed is the first step in the treatment plan. Keeping the lines of communication open and being willing to work with your therapist is the first step to healing your body, your mind, and your spirit. Consistency is the key to overall healing."

Pump You Up!

Exercise, a good diet, and taking care of the body beautiful aren't the only ways you can stay pumped. Start reading magazines and books that pump you up. I highly recommend *Figure Magazine* and *Heart and Soul Magazine*. *Figure* is a magazine designed with size 12 and over in mind. The articles are fresh, the writers are hip, and the clothes are sexy. The features celebrate the total plus woman: mind, body, and soul. *Heart and Soul* is designed to keep in tune with healthy living for women of all sizes. Moreover, through its use of cover models (from size 6 to size 22), it shows the world that healthy doesn't necessarily come in small packages. (Also check out the Just My Size styles on the Internet at www.jms.com.)

That's the key! Feeling good about yourself and not needing to be validated by society at large. Resist the urge to put on a cover-up. After all, if thin women can get away with wearing revealing outfits (with nothing to reveal to speak of), why can't we? Besides, clothes look far more appealing when they hug the curves and hint at the possibility of DANGER. This is your time to feel good, look good, and know it. Walk down the street with your head held high, switch your butt, and show the world you are proud of your "bounce to the ounce."

WEDDING OVERLOAD

Even though getting married is a wonderful time in life, it's also a time when you seem to become consumed with planning and talking about your wedding. Before that happens, declare a "wedding free" day. What I mean by that is set aside a day in which neither you, your fiancé, your family, nor your friends will discuss your wedding plans. After all, before you got engaged, you had a life! I know all your friends and family mean well. A wedding is something to talk about. The problem is when it becomes the focus of all conversation.

A wedding is only the celebration of the joining of two lives. The ceremony just makes it official—whether you're married in St. Patrick's Cathedral or city hall. It's your life after the wedding that matters. So while it's lovely to discuss dresses and flowers, take a time out. Give your mind a rest! Take the time to go out on a date with your fiancé instead of getting together to discuss the wedding. Perhaps you could take a nostalgic trip to where you first met, go antique shopping, take hikes, or just go to your favorite restaurant. Spend time together just being yourselves. Granted, you have the wedding on your mind, but before the wedding plans came you were a couple, and you will still be a couple after the wedding.

If all else fails, go shopping! Remember, this is still part of your wedding-free zone, so go into some of your favorite clothing boutiques and look for some R & R clothes. Maybe a new pair of jeans, a dress, shorts, or a shirt. Venture into the many new stores that actually have fashionable clothing in your size. Experiment in new colors and patterns you've never had the nerve to put on. Be brave and buy that short skirt for work. You know the one—the one that up until now you thought was too daring to wear.

DISABLED DIVAS

I have multiple sclerosis (MS), so I am especially sensitive to the needs of the disabled. I am very aware of how your life changes when you have wheels or live on crutches (those third and fourth "legs"). Suddenly you become more conscious of your body and how people look at you. Due to MS, I use a crutch to help me walk distances. As a result, I know how embarrassing it is when people stare. But the man in my life doesn't see them at all, even when he's tripping over them. He loves me as I am. And I'm sure when your groom is standing at the altar, all he sees is the most beautiful woman in the world.

Here are some things to remember:

- Make and keep regular appointments with your doctor.

- Never forget to take your medication, no matter how busy you are.

- If you belong to a support group, don't forget to go. A support group isn't just about being there when you're down, it's about sharing your good feelings with others as well.

- The MS Society has a newsletter and quarterly magazine that I read cover to cover. It's filled with information on current studies, therapies, classifieds, and inspirational stories. There are many other national organizations for diabetes, epilepsy, lupus, etc. Get a subscription if you don't already have one.

- For those of you who use assistive equipment, be sure to discuss your logistical concerns with your wedding day venue well ahead of time. Don't wait until the last minute; you'll bring on undue stress.

- Talk to your physician about massage therapy.

- If you're diabetic, consult your doctor before scheduling an appointment for a pedicure to limit any risks.

- Listen to your body. Take breaks as often as needed.

- Ask for help. Make sure you keep your fiancé in the loop.

- Schedule your appointments carefully. Don't try to pack everything into one day.

- Don't fill up your whole day with wedding plans. Take a walk. Watch your favorite soap. Call a friend.

- Relax and enjoy being the center of attention.

Beautiful Celebrations

Now for the party! This is the part of your wedding where you need to consider the other special people involved in your big day—your bridesmaids, other attendants, your family, and your guests. Making the day meet your expectations as well as their comfort requires planning. This chapter will help you put together all the details that make the day special for everyone. And since money is a major factor for most brides, let's start there.

PLANNING AND BUDGET

I'm about to ask you and your fiancé some questions. Whether you have dreamed all your life about your wedding or never thought twice about it, this approach will help you decide what you really want, organize your plans, and catch any details you might have missed.

Both you and your fiancé should answer these questions, and I want you to take an unusual approach. Think about the biggest celebration you could ever imagine. Don't worry about the budget. Focus only on what you would have for your wedding if money were no object. Now before you panic, let me explain.

By no means am I telling you to go into debt so you can have the grandest, most unaffordable wedding possible. Rather, I want you to be honest with yourself about what you want. All too often a bride will say she wants a small wedding just to save money. If that's what you truly want, great! But be sure you're not just saying that because you feel you have to.

Too many times I have seen a wedding scenario start out small, then suddenly take on a life of its own. Guest lists that start with one hundred people quickly jump to two hundred. Seasonable flower arrangements give way to expensive tropicals and exotic styles, and simple pew bows expand to flowers and votive candles. I could go on, but you get the picture.

It is far easier to scale a large wedding down than to upgrade a small one. Plus think of the frustration, stress, and expense you will save by being honest with yourself and your fiancé about what you want. If you plan carefully and shop around, having the type of wedding you want doesn't necessarily preclude affordability. Wedding specialists can offer you advice on alternatives to include style, substance, and panache without sacrificing your wallet in the process.

So take some time to answer the following questions honestly (apart from each other). Then compare your answers to decide what will work best for both of you.

1. The style of your wedding is your most important question. How do you envision the day? Will it

be formal, semi-formal, dressy casual, casual, or come as you are? (Remember, these questions are designed to elicit your true feelings, so be honest.)

2. Do you have a fantasy about your wedding? What would be the ideal wedding day for you?

3. What is your favorite time of year? Is there a certain time of day that you prefer?

4. What type of service do you want for your reception? Do you prefer a laid-back buffet or the formality of white-glove service?

5. What are some of your favorite foods? Are you a steak and potatoes person? Do you like to try a wide variety of ethnic cuisines, or are you into a specific type of cuisine like Thai, French, or Northern Italian?

6. As far as beverages are concerned, do you prefer beer, wine, tropical drinks, or soft drinks?

7. What are some of your favorite colors?

8. What are your favorite flowers? Why do you like them and how do they make you feel? Do they evoke certain memories for you?

9. What kind of music do you like? Are you a country western buff, or are Mozart and Brahms more your speed? When you venture out to see a live show, is it old school rap, hip-hop, golden oldies, big bands, stringed quartets, folk music, or jazz that moves you?

10. As far as your pictures are concerned, do you want the formality of posed portraits, or would you prefer the less formal documentary or photojournalistic style? How do you feel about having pictures taken? Are you a "ham" for the camera or "camera shy"? If you are camera shy, how and why did you come to be that way?

Now let's do some planning based on your answers.

Where

Wedding locations fall into two areas, indoor and outdoor. On-site, indoor locations (a church, catering halls, country clubs, hotels, etc.) have all the services you need for your wedding. This type of service is perfect for today's busy brides because someone else is taking care of the details. An indoor wedding is by far the type most often chosen by couples. It offers insurance against the elements and allows you to plan your wonderful day down to the last detail. An indoor location also means you are usually working within a set décor, but it does not mean your venue can't reflect your style and taste.

Off-site, outdoor weddings are beautiful because nature provides a perfectly balanced landscape of color to make your event come alive. Here are some suggestions:

• The beach.

- A city park.

- A country inn.

- A picturesque valley.

- The grounds of a mansion or an historical home.

- Someone's backyard.

While outdoor settings provide much of their own décor and ambience, they also require some unique planning to run smoothly. You will need to take into account the following issues:

- Check the weather for the time of year and the location of your wedding. For instance, an outdoor wedding in Arizona is not a good idea in the summer. Likewise, a tropical outdoor wedding in Florida during hurricane season would be a disaster.

- Be sure to order a tent in case of bad weather. Be sure you know where the tent will be set up on your site and what restrictions may exist for the site. You should also be aware of the difference between a tent and a canopy. A canopy is similar to a tent; however, it doesn't usually come with walls, and it doesn't require professional installation. It is usually secured from an existing structure. A tent, on the other hand, is free standing and comes with walls. It is installed professionally for most events, which gives you some assurance of its sturdiness. Significant factors such as rain or wind should also be considered when planning an outdoor event. You will want to reserve an alternate site in case the weather deteriorates even beyond tent use.

- If you plan to have dancing, order a dance floor.

- Outdoor wedding rentals should be arranged at least four to six months prior to the event. Stay in contact with the rental service and verify who will be setting up the equipment on the day of your wedding. For weddings on a public beach, at a park, or in a public garden, make reservations and get the proper permits. In some cases your caterer or florist can be of service to you. If they specialize in off-site events, they may already be familiar with the requirements of the location you are considering.

- Consider the logistics of how your guests will get to your event and where they will park. Consider any long walking distances for elderly or disabled guests, and what assistance they might need. If you're getting married at a home, you'll need to arrange for extra guest parking. Neighbors are often willing to lend a hand; ask if their driveways can be used for overflow parking.

- If your location is a private site or home, you will need to consider the restroom facilities. If the wedding is small enough, existing restrooms may be sufficient. In many cases, however, the facilities may be insufficient, or worse still, nonexistent. If this is the case, you will need to rent some Port-

O-Lets or Port-O-Sans. You need not consider this tacky; they are set up like real bathrooms. You should, however, make sure they are well-placed and accessible.

- If you are planning to have your ceremony at one location and your reception at another, try to keep the travel time between sites down to thirty minutes or less. Both you and your guests will appreciate it.

For more wonderful tips on planning an outdoor wedding, contact the American Rental Association at 1 (800) 334-2177, or online at www.ararental.org.

When

Everyone has a favorite season, and the best season for a wedding is definitely a matter of taste. But many people do not realize that it is also a matter of cost.

Spring is the most popular season for weddings, but it is also the most expensive. If you've always dreamed of being a June bride, you will need to book a catering hall eighteen months in advance (or even earlier depending on the popularity of the facility). On the other hand, if you're willing to get married in early spring, you can save money and still be a spring bride.

Summer is a 50/50 wedding season depending upon where you live. In areas where the three H's (hot, hazy, and humid) are a part of the everyday vocabulary, you must plan for an indoor and well air-conditioned wedding. But in cooler climates, summer evenings lend themselves to beautiful outdoor weddings.

As the lushness of summer greenery gives way to a cornucopia of vibrant fall colors, autumn's comfortable temperatures provide a wonderful setting for a wedding. Catering halls and wedding facilities begin to slow down, particularly after Indian summer, and you may be able to find reasonable deals for your reception without sacrificing style.

A white wedding in winter can warm the cockles of your heart without burning a lot of your cash. Winter is traditionally a slow time for catering halls, many of which offer special prices for weddings.

And finally, a few general notes about seasons. Holidays are always an expensive time for a wedding. It may seem very romantic to be married on St. Valentine's Day, but you will pay premium prices for the privilege. Flowers, services, and sites are all more expensive on holidays because of high demand. Valentine's Day and Christmas are the most expensive holidays to plan around. You will also pay more for seasonal items such as flowers if your wedding is not scheduled when they are normally available.

Who

This is a very intricate element of wedding planning. The number of guests will directly affect your budget and possibly the setting for your wedding. Both you and your fiancé should make a list and then review the lists together for overlap and appropriateness.

As you plan the final guest list, keep personalities in mind. Is your list filled with people who love lingering conversation? If so, plan an event that gives them plenty of time to visit. Or perhaps you have a real party crowd that needs a fast paced program to hold their interest. If your list is a mixture of generations, you might want to consider ways to bridge the gap.

Another aspect of your guest list is that of compatibility. Many of us have divorced parents, relatives, or friends whom we want to have attend this most special occasion. If you can comfortably speak to them about their preferences, do so; if not, do yourself a favor and place them at separate tables. In such cases, it is easier not to flirt with disaster.

And while we're on the subject of who, let's consider your wedding party. Be prepared to be on everyone's "Most Wanted" list. Friends or relatives may simply presume they should be bridesmaids. Your mother may suddenly start pointing out relatives who should be included: those you know, those you can't remember for the life of you, and those you wish you didn't know. Nevertheless, you have the final say.

I'm a firm believer that less is more. I have seen wedding parties so large they boggled the mind. So while you may want to have those who are close to you in your wedding party, you need not include everyone. If your guests have endured the entrance of 14 bridesmaids (not including the flower girl), your own entrance will be anti-climatic. Remember, the highpoint of the day comes when you leave your guests breathless at the sight of your radiance, not relieved that the "train" has finally passed.

Still, if a small bridal party is not an option, there are ways to cope with size. Fashion and style aspects discussed in the following sections can come to your rescue and leave your guests breathlessly anticipating your arrival.

Wedding Themes

A wedding theme is the result of your artistic expression—the vision you've created for your wedding. When described this way it may seem like a monumental task, but it's really quite simple.

Your theme should be based on something personal and special to you and the groom. For example, a couple that met at a Halloween party incorporated a masquerade theme into their wedding. The wedding was formal, but the guests carried masks made famous at Truman Capote's Black and White Ball. Or maybe you have a shared passion (i.e., sports team or hobby) you want to celebrate.

Wedding themes aren't just for the wealthy; they can be

done on a budget. Through careful planning you can have the wedding of your dreams. All you need is your imagination and enough time to plan things carefully. Here are a few tips:

- Once you've decided on a theme, begin looking into vendors, wholesalers, and retailers where you can buy your supplies at a discount.

- Even if you're not the most craft-oriented person in the world, it would be prudent to check out craft projects that you can do yourself to save money.

- Talk to your catering hall manager to see what items they can procure for your theme, and if they can be included in your wedding package.

Contracts

Before we move on to the specifics of the wedding party, there is one last but very important point to discuss under Planning and Budget. As you deal with the various aspects of your wedding, you should ask about each professional's (or service organization's) contract. Just as you did when ordering your gown and arranging for your beauty salon, ask about price, payment schedules, cancellation policies, and special pricing for large orders, etc.

Now, on to the specifics.

ATTENDANTS

Mothers

Traditionally, mothers have the privilege of choosing their own attire. However, many mothers face the same full-figure issues you do. Don't be afraid to share what you have learned with this most important person.

Bridesmaids

Bridesmaid's dresses are the stuff of folklore. Where else can a bridesmaid experience the thrill of victory (a dress she loves and will wear again) or the sheer agony of defeat (a dress she will burn at the first opportunity)?

Your bridesmaids are the women you hold nearest and dearest to your heart. Make sure they shine. I guarantee they won't overshadow you; they'll only add to your glorious illumination. Who knows? They might want you to be a bridesmaid one day. Stack the odds in your favor and make them look good; you just might avoid a tangerine satin nightmare in the future.

Choose a dress reflective of your personal style. Whether you go with a long or short length, make sure the style is flattering, elegant, sexy, and affordable. Most of all, be sure it's a dress that can be worn again. Use what you have learned about body shapes and style to make each person look her best.

When thinking about the bridesmaid's dresses, you can use several approaches:

1. Identical dresses in the same color and fabric (the most typical and homogeneous approach).

2. Identical dresses in different colors.

3. Different dress styles in the same fabric and color.

4. Different dress styles in different fabrics, but the same color.

When going with identical dresses (i.e., color and style), try to still include something distinctive about each bridesmaid: her jewelry, hair accessories, or gloves.

If you want identical dresses in different colors, choose colors within the same color family. In any event, make sure the colors you choose are in keeping with the colors of your wedding.

In the case of both No. 3 and No. 4, this is a complete judgment call. In most weddings, it is the maid of honor who wears a different style dress with the rest wearing the same style gown. To keep it under control, try choosing similar dresses with different style elements. For instance, if you choose an A-line style dress, you can have it made sleeveless, with a V-neck, strapless, or with a halter.

Just like your wedding gown, body shape, fabric, and cost are important elements to consider when selecting bridesmaids' dresses. Unless you are purchasing their dresses, keep your bridesmaids' checkbooks in mind as you choose the most flattering styles and fabrics. Also keep in mind that you will need to begin this search at least eight to ten months before the wedding.

Here's an idea. Have a "bridesmaids' party." That's right, a bridesmaids' party! It can be a slumber party or a luncheon—either one would be fine. Just invite them over for an afternoon or night of girl talk and goodies. If you have a couple of junior bridesmaids, invite their mothers as well. Ask each of them to bring their favorite fashion magazine, and in the meantime, pick up a couple of bridal magazines or brochures to have on hand. Talk about fashion design. Get their opinions with an informal survey. Have each bridesmaid pick a gown she likes and write it down. Take note of the cost range they can afford, from high to low. After you've giggled and laughed for a while, take out the old tape measure. If one or two of the girls are a little too shy to share their measurements, elect yourself as the measurement keeper. Once you have all the measurements, you are now in possession of a blueprint to aid you in making them look their best.

Teenage Bridesmaids

If you were a full-figured girl yourself, you'd probably rather forget the teen years. Fortunately for to-day's plus-size teens, there is a lot more support, understanding, and most importantly, fashion choice, than ever before. It's not necessary to automatically pick out a "skinny" dress in a larger size. There are many dresses made to fit and flatter a fuller frame. Accentuate the positive—within reason of course.

Get input from the teenage bridesmaids' parents. I know we automatically ask moms, but fathers should have a say in what their daughters wear, too. After all, these are those weird in-between years when they're not little girls and not grown women. It's up to you to find the equilibrium.

A number of young plus-size women's cups runneth over, as mine did when I was a teenager. To be hon-est, even before I was a teenager. In fifth grade I was already a B-cup, so you know how much fun recess was for me. In junior high I was in a C-cup and a DD-cup by the time I graduated high school. So what did my parents do when it came time for me to dress up? They made sure I was tastefully dressed to look my age.

A friend of mine named Denise Nelson arranged for her daughters (ages 13 and 15 respectively) to be an exquisite part of her wedding. To make them feel special and beautiful, she chose two very flattering dress-es—and they made lovely bridesmaids. If you're planning to have a special teenager in your wedding, you would do well to check out sites like www.sydneyscloset.com or www.sowhatif.com for stylish dresses for weddings and proms. Another terrific site to explore is www.micheleweston.com. Michele Weston of MJW Style Media/Selling Style LLC is a motivational writer and fashion diva for full-grown divas and divas-in-training.

Child Attendants

Most of us have a little person in mind for our wedding. Whether it's your own child, a niece or nephew, a godchild, or a special friend's son or daughter, children are a wonderful addition to any wedding party (provided they don't steal the show—which they usually do).

When selecting the attire for child attendants, you would do well to keep cost in mind. While many parents would love to have their child participate, if the cost is too high they'll regrettably have to bow out. If you find an outfit that you love and it's expensive, you may want to offer to help offset the cost, or if possible, pay for it yourself.

You will also need to make sure that their attire is in keeping with the rest of the bridal party since they will precede the bride. Above all, I cannot emphasize enough that although children should look the part, they should still look like children.

CEREMONIES

As I stated earlier, the ceremony is the most important part of your wedding. It is the time in which you and your groom profess your love to each other, to God, to your friends and family, and to the world at large. The ceremony makes your commitment to each other legal and binding, and should be marked with the respect and reverence it deserves.

There are four basic types of ceremonies:

Religious   A member of the clergy officiates. This includes a Pastor, Reverend, Priest, Bishop, Rabbi, or any other ordained minister.

Interfaith   This is when there are two individuals of different faiths officiating in the capacity of their faith. For example, a rabbi and priest, or a priest and a minister.

Civil   This is where a judge, mayor, or captain (when at sea) officiates.

Spiritual   This ceremony focuses on humanity as a whole instead of focusing on religious doctrines or beliefs. The same officials as those listed above (as well as other government officials) can officiate, but the bride and groom can write and perform their own ceremony.

No matter which ceremony you choose, make sure your official clearly understands what you want. If you would like to have members of your family read scripture during the ceremony, have a favorite hymn performed, or if you want to incorporate your own vows, make sure the official is aware of this so adjustments can be made. Be open to suggestions based on the official's past experience.

Also, make sure that you are clear on whether or not you are going to have a traditional or a nontraditional setting. Will you walk down the aisle with your father, or is your mother giving you away? Perhaps you are walking down the aisle alone. How many people will be in your party? Iron out details like these well before the wedding.

Depending upon where you hold your ceremony, envision the setting you desire. Maybe you want to have votive candles at the entrance of the church and tulle adorning each pew. Or perhaps you want a trellis covered with roses where you and the groom will stand. Before you start dreaming up wonderful ideas, however, make sure they are, in fact, realistic. If you're getting married in a church, there could be regulations against certain embellishments. Make sure you speak to your official to see what applies to you.

Getting married is an intimate experience, so make sure your guests can feel close to you as well. If you're getting married in a large outdoor venue, you can have the chairs set up amphitheater style so everyone can see the proceedings. You will also need to pay attention to the acoustics, making sure you're not only seen, but heard.

If you are incorporating special items into your ceremony (poetry readings, choirs, "jumping the broom," etc.), you may want to have a program printed that includes a list of the participants. It could also mention those special friends and family members who are absent or have passed away.

Music

When choosing the music for your ceremony, you need to remember that music is a powerful force that creates a mood. So as you plan the musical prelude for your wedding, give some thought to the type of mood you're setting—whether it's provided by a live band or a recording.

Here are some classical and contemporary music standards:

- Ave Maria

- Wagner's Wedding March

- Brandenburg Concertos, by Bach

- Love Theme, by Tchaikovsky

- Pomp and Circumstance No 4, by Elgar

- Vivaldi's Spring (Four Seasons)

- Water Music, by Handel

- Mendelssohn's Wedding March

- The Wedding Song, by Kenny G

- Just the Two of Us, by Grover Washington, Jr.

- Unforgettable, by Nat King Cole

- The First Time Ever I Saw Your Face, by Roberta Flack

- Selections offered by your church's choir or a soloist.

Flowers

Who could ever forget the first time their love gave them flowers and how it made them feel. This is the feeling you want to incorporate into your wedding decor.

While flowers are beautiful, they can also prove to be very expensive: from your wedding bouquet right down to the centerpieces on each table. However, you can make choices that will provide you with beautiful arrangements that are still cost-effective.

The first step is to find a reputable florist, and the time to start looking is up to twelve months before the wedding. Get personal recommendations. Take the time for a leisurely visit to several shops in person. Are their arrangements ordinary, creative, or spectacular? Is business brisk or slow? Remember, you want someone who can be creative and stylish within an allotted budget.

Once you find a florist that fits your needs, make sure you take the designers a picture of your gown or pictures of arrangements you like. If your florist is going to be designing the arrangements for both the ceremony and the reception sites, make sure the designers see the site so they will have a better overall idea of how everything is to be set up.

Bouquets

If you are going with fresh flowers for your bouquet and your attendants' bouquets, you will want to make sure that the bouquets are both beautiful and practical. While we all love flowers, carrying around a large bouquet of flowers for several hours can test the strength of even a die-hard flower lover. What I suggest is that you order an arrangement that is big enough to be seen without making your wrist feel like it's going to fall off.

Types of Bridal Bouquets include:

Heart-Shaped   A bouquet in the shape of a heart.

Cascade   A bouquet that falls forward.

Teardrop   A cascade in the shape of an inverted teardrop.

Round/Nosegay   A round, tight bouquet of flowers.

Arm Bouquet   A loose bouquet held across the arm.

Hand-Tied   A bouquet held together by a ribbon, usually with visible stems.

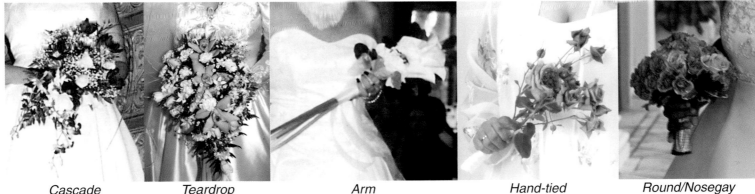

Cascade   *Teardrop*   *Arm*   *Hand-tied*   *Round/Nosegay*

Wee Bee Country Florist in Amityville, New York, has been a staple in that village for over ten years. Owner Bob Perillo is a talented floral designer and someone brides past and present have come to rely on to create beautiful arrangements in any price range. Mr. Perillo states, "Forget the mother's corsage or the bridesmaids' flowers, the bride's flowers are the most important arrangement at the wedding. Yet they should not take anything away from the bride, which is why I try to stay away from big overpowering arrangements.

"I particularly prefer a cascading bouquet for full-figured brides. It's a very beautiful bouquet as it lengthens the line, but it doesn't take attention away from the bride."

Here are some of Bob Perillo's tips:

- Once you decide on a date and set a budget, start shopping around for florists (at least six months to a year before the wedding).

- Find out how far in advance they book weddings and how many weddings they do at a time. If they do more than six weddings a day, you can't be guaranteed a floral designer will be working on your event.

- Find out how far in advance they make their bouquets.

- Remember, even if you're on a budget, order early and make payments throughout the time period. Some florists are willing to work with you on a payment plan.

Bridesmaids' Bouquets

There are many ways to personalize the bouquets of your attendants. The maid or matron of honor can carry a copy of the bridal bouquet, only smaller. Bridesmaids can carry similar bouquets but in different colors. For a more relaxed or less formal wedding, the bridesmaids can carry hand bouquets tied with ribbons.

Groom's and Groomsmen's Boutonnieres

Even though a lot of attention is given to the bridal flowers, the groom and his groomsmen deserve equal attention. "The boutonnieres should be lovely, tasteful, and compliment the bride's bouquet," says Bob Perillo.

Centerpiece Arrangements

My advice as far as centerpieces are concerned is that you don't need very expensive flowers in order to create a beautiful arrangement. Technically, you don't need flowers as centerpieces at all. There is a way to combine both elegance and economics. Consider alternative arrangements like fruit whimsically arranged, meaningful keepsakes or photos, or rose petals scattered on the tables. If you choose to go with flowers, keep in mind that floral containers can be more expensive than the flowers themselves; be selective. Above all, be mindful of height. After all, you put a lot of thought into the seating arrangements so your guests could socialize. Your guests should be able to see either over or under the centerpieces. If you prefer tall arrangements, they should use narrow pedestals that allow seated guests to see past them.

Once you've determined the shop you want to use for your floral arrangements, ask for details: flower types, deposit requirements, total cost, and cancellation policies. These should all be included in a signed agreement.

Here are a few questions that need answers before you sign on the dotted line:

1. Does your florist charge a consulting fee for the first meeting?

2. How do bouquets vary in shape and price?

3. Is there a price list you can take home?

4. Do they have books showing other arrangements they've prepared for prior weddings?

5. Have they worked at your wedding site in the past?

6. Will they visit the ceremony and reception sites in order to get an idea of how the flowers should be arranged?

7. Will you receive a sample bridal bouquet?

8. What flowers will be in season for your wedding?

9. If the flowers you order aren't available, what substitutions can be made and at what cost?

10. If you have a very large order, what concessions can be made regarding additional items, such as a throw-away bouquet at no additional charge?

11. Who will be responsible for the on-site setup? At what time will the flowers be delivered, and at what location?

12. How long will the setup take?

13. If items from the ceremony are to be moved to the reception site, will the florist help move them, and at what charge?

14. Will your florist preserve the bouquet or recommend ways that you can do it yourself?

15. What will be the total cost of your order? Will they set up a payment schedule for you? Is there a policy for payments?

Once you have all of these questions answered satisfactorily, you'll be ready to proceed with the contract.

Menus

Now it's time to talk about the reception. If you are having your reception in a centralized location, you were probably given a menu from which you could choose. Easy! In addition, most receptions halls provide white glove service. However, very few offer buffet style meals. If your reception is being held at an off-site location, you will have much more freedom in determining the menu and service.

When developing your menu, it's best to keep your choices simple. Perhaps grilled chicken instead of filet mignon en croûte. This will allow for the even cooking and presentation of your main course. Once you've decided on your main course, you can plan your side dishes around it.

Keep in mind that it's not necessary to have a traditional sit-down dinner. There are many alternatives to consider. For example:

Cocktail Reception

This type of reception focuses on appetizers, crudités, fresh fruit, cheeses, and crackers. These can be presented "butler style" (which means served by waiters), or buffet style. Along with the food, one can have champagne, various alcoholic and nonalcoholic drinks, and coffee.

Wedding Brunch

This type of reception is easy and elegant. It's perfect for spring, summer, and early fall weddings since it is easy to set up outdoors. The menu would typically include mimosas (orange juice with sparkling wine or champagne), an assortment of quick breads and morning pastries (such as croissants, muffins, and scones), fresh fruit in season, tea and coffee, and, of course, the wedding cake.

Tea Reception

The idea of taking tea in the afternoon is one that is associated with an era of Victorian elegance gone by. Today you can take advantage of this by having an afternoon tea reception. Usually taken around 3:00 p.m., you can offer your guests tea sandwiches, canapés, scones, crumpets, pastries, fruit, and wedding cake. For beverages you can offer sherry, sparkling water, punch, and (of course) Earl Grey Tea.

Wedding Luncheon

In any season, wedding luncheons are classic. Since they involve much less work and preparation than a sit-down dinner, guests are treated to a relaxed style of elegance. Luncheon menus are usually served in courses. Depending on the season, the first course can be a Mesclun salad, chilled bisque, or a warming soup. The main course should fit the season and would be followed by wedding cake, an assortment of fruits in season, or sorbets. The beverages could be an assortment of sparkling wines, Cabernet Sauvignons, mineral water, punch, soft drinks, tea, and coffee.

Dessert Buffet

Another option for a reception is a dessert buffet. This is a beautiful way to combine all your favorite pies, pastries, and cookies with your wedding cake. The dessert buffet is usually served with champagne punch, champagne, sparkling wines, soft drinks, tea, and coffee.

Buffet Dinner

This type of reception is truly a loosening of the tie that usually goes with a sit-down affair. Guests are encouraged to mingle with one another while sampling from the table. A buffet dinner is also a great way to incorporate a theme. For instance, if you want a feeling of Island Carnival, you can choose a menu of plantains, miniature beef patties, Johnny cakes, and jerk chicken—just to name a few. Or if you want a southern feel, maybe a menu of southern fried chicken and cornbread with peach cobbler. The combinations are endless. Give it your personal touch or mix things up a bit—it's completely up to you. Depending on the number of people you invite, a buffet can be less expensive; however, if you're planning a large wedding, a sit down meal may be more economical since a buffet requires more staff to service and replenish the food trays, dinnerware, and cutlery.

Rehearsal Dinner

There are so many details to keep straight during the course of planning a wedding that some get lost in the shuffle. One of those little details is the rehearsal dinner. Rosa Campbell is someone who knows all about keeping a lot of little details straight. "All the planning for the wedding has been completed, you're down to your last two weeks, and you remember the rehearsal dinner! All your finances have been exhausted. What should you do? A restaurant is way too expensive."

Rosa's Tips:

Location   Find an ideal location such as your home, your parents' or in-laws' homes, a friend's place, or a church that won't cost you extra money.

Menu   Choose a simple menu—one or two main entrées, vegetables, salads, breads, and a light dessert. Limit the beverage choices: a refreshing punch would do nicely.

Preparation   This menu could be catered professionally, or friends and family could do the cooking.

The Cake

You have planned all the details of your wedding down to the letter. The dress is perfect, the reception site is grand, and you are at your most beautiful. Still, after all is said and done, the one thing guests are sure to remember is the cake. The wedding cake is the highlight of a reception. It's a memory many guests carry around for years.

I remember attending an unfortunate outdoor wedding where I watched the cake melt before my eyes.

I don't remember what color the bridesmaids wore, but I do remember that the food was awful and the cake was as disappointing to the taste as it was to the eye. So a lot is riding on your choice of a baker for your wedding cake.

Before you sit down with a caterer or a baker, give some consideration to these factors:

1. What time of year is the wedding?

2. Will it be outdoors or indoors?

3. How many guests will you need to serve?

4. What preference do you have as far as icing is concerned?

5. Do you want the cake presented on tiers with columns or on a cake stand?

6. Does the baker use fresh flowers for decorating or will the flowers be made of gum paste, fondant, or buttercream?

All of these factors affect the type of cake you decide to have. For instance, if you're having an outdoor wedding and you love whipped cream icing, you will need to have an alternative since whipped cream will literally disintegrate outdoors.

Here are a few terms you need to know to help you when you talk to your baker/caterer:

Buttercream — This is the most common type of icing. It is a combination of high quality butter and sugar. This type of icing is commonly used for its stability.

Fondant — This is a confection icing that is rolled out and placed over the layers of cake for a smooth finish. There is a great difference in taste depending on whether your baker uses domestic or English fondant. I prefer to make my own, but if I had to choose, English fondant is of far better quality.

Ganache — This is a combination of chocolate, cream, and butter that is poured over cake layers and allowed to set.

Royal Icing — This is a cooked icing that dries to a hard finish. It is usually reserved for decorations such as flowers or ribbons.

Marzipan — This is an almond paste that can be formed and colored to resemble flowers, fruits, or leaves.

The choice of wedding cake flavors and fillings is endless. You might consider having a nontraditional cake like carrot cake, cheesecake, or Jamaican black cake. Another option is the Croquembouche, which is constructed of cream puffs and fashioned to resemble a tree. Guests "pluck" the cream puffs from the "tree."

Once you have selected the type of cake you want, be sure to go over the contract with the baker carefully to be sure there is no miscommunication with regards to what you ordered. Do not assume anything.

BEAUTIFUL CELEBRATIONS

Rosa Campbell, a professional event planner who recently expanded into personal/wedding event planning, concurs. She states, "I was helping a friend out for a wedding and she asked me to wait for the cake to be delivered, since every other detail had been attended to. Not only did the cake arrive later than originally stated in the contract, it wasn't the cake the bride ordered to match her colors of cream and gold—it was black (chocolate) and white."

Don't let this happen to you. Check and double check so you get exactly what you paid for.

Beautiful Memories

Throw the ten pounds the camera adds out the window. You have more important things to worry about. It's important to feel beautiful because it's your essence the camera will reflect, not your chin or thighs. I'll be honest—even I have fallen victim to trying to create the perfect pose. You know the one: it's when you simultaneously hold your stomach in, stick out your neck, and turn your head on an angle to get a thinner shot. What happens is that you wind up looking unnatural, or worse . . . constipated! So exhale and relax. Let the photographer worry about the angles. He's a professional; it's his job. Your only job is to smile!

According to Jake Mincey of Precise Creations, "It's important for a subject to feel comfortable. If they're uncomfortable, it shows in the pictures. That's why I like to take my time and ease into the atmosphere."

CHOOSING A PHOTOGRAPHER

Before you let your fingers do the walking, stop and take a deep breath. Do you really want to trust an unknown photographer you found in the yellow pages with the most important pictures of your life?

Here are some tips to help you in making this important decision.

- Ask to see the photographer's portfolio to determine the range of subjects with which he or she has worked.

- Ask for recommendations from friends and family.

You need your photographer to be an experienced professional who appreciates the beauty of a full-figured woman and knows how to photograph her. Oleg Vertiniskii of Studio B1 Photography has worked with brides of all sizes. With a degree in architectural design, Oleg is a master of form and composition. He states, "Full-figured women are deeply appreciated by millions of men in the USA and around the globe—including me. I've met a lot of men who love large women, and I'll always remember a groom, actually a husband at the moment, who was crying while looking at the wedding photographs of his full-figured wife that I'd just printed for them and kept saying, 'Isn't she beautiful? I love the way she looks in these pictures.'

"On the other hand, under the influence of the common belief among women that skinny is beautiful (which is thrown at us from just about every commercial or printed advertisement), most brides want to look slimmer. They want to be the stars of their special day, and most stars on TV and in the movies look like they never eat!

"Consequently I, as the photographer, have to satisfy two conflicting requests: the groom loves the bride just the way she is, so that's how he wants to see her in photographs; but the bride thinks skinnier is better, and she wants me to slim her down a size or two. You wouldn't believe how many beautiful women look at themselves in the mirror and think how ugly they are.

"As a result, I have developed some lighting, composition, and cropping techniques that make both newlyweds happy. The approach I've developed over the years of shooting full-figured brides (actually, this applies to most brides I've worked with) satisfies the desires of the groom and the bride: the bride looks slimmer overall, but the single parts of her body look as plump as they can without distorting that slimmed down look."

Oleg offers the following formula for "full-figured photo" success to all photographers:

LIGHTING

- Avoid broad lighting. It makes the face of the subject appear wider than it actually is. Broad lighting is when the light illuminates the side of the face that is turned toward the camera. If you use a "built-in" or "mounted-on-the-camera flash," this is what you get—broad lighting. If you use broad lighting you'll get flat, wide, oily faces in most of your pictures, and I don't want to be there when the bride takes the first look at your finished product.

- Use short lighting as much as possible. It makes the face of the subject appear narrower. Short (or narrow) lighting is when the light illuminates the part of the face that is turned away from the camera. I usually use a strobe light with a soft box positioned at about 30–40 degrees. It gives you nice soft shadows and some diffused light bouncing from the walls and the ceiling to fill those shadowed areas a little bit so they are not too dark.

- If your subject's face is not wide but there is a double chin to take care of, use butterfly lighting, which is when you position the light directly in front of the subject's face and move it up until you get the shadows under the nose and the chin. It will cover the double chin and as an added benefit, will make a short nose appear much longer.

- Rembrandt lighting (which is a combination of short and butterfly lighting) will slim your subject down dramatically, but be careful here. It will also emphasize all skin imperfections such as acne, for the angle of the light is very low and the shadows are very long.

COMPOSITION

The rules of composition are an independent topic, and are so large that I cannot discuss them in much detail here. (However, you should follow the rules of composition until you know when or how to break them.)

- Crop your photographs properly when shooting; it will save you time and effort down the road.

- Symmetric, centered composition tends to make your subject appear larger and stiff.

- Move your subject away from the center of your image and create some additional space in the picture. It may look like a wasted area, but it will serve your purpose; it will make your subject look smaller and the whole picture will be more interesting.

- By cropping out some parts of your subject's body, you will slim your model down considerably.

- I prefer portrait (vertical) formats when shooting full-figured brides; it makes the subject appear leaner and adds some energy to the shoot. Landscape (horizontal) formats make people look larger and will suck the energy from your pictures. It's only appropriate for shooting large groups of people.

- Get rid of all distracting elements in your picture by zooming in, standing closer, or picking a different shooting angle.

- Use furniture or anything else in the room to block the parts of the bride's body that are irrelevant or make her look larger.

- Be careful with your view angle. Shooting down on the bride will hide her double chin and the wrinkles on her neck and make her body appear smaller in relation to her head. Shooting up while crouching down will exaggerate the bride's body and reveal the areas that will not complement the subject at all. If it's a full-length portrait, an eye-level view makes the bride look shorter. Move your camera down to approximately breast level to indicate height more accurately and make your subject look slimmer.

POSING

- As a rule, I personally prefer to move myself around the bride and groom while shooting. Subconsciously, people don't like being moved and pushed around, and if you do it to them, you'll end up with some stiff, frozen bodies with fake smiles on their faces angrily looking into your camera. If you really need to move and pose them, make sure you do it in a very polite manner. Don't do it more than once for every new position, and try to make them believe it was their own idea. Demonstrate the poses you want yourself rather than giving orders to your subjects. Don't adjust your camera and equipment too much when your subjects are ready, it will make them definitely uneasy and maybe even angry.

- When people move, their facial muscles relax and it results in a more natural look. It also reduces the number of their wrinkles. The body tonus increases when the muscles tighten up, improving the body's shape. So give them a shoot while they're on the move: you'll be surprised how much difference it makes. In general, people look happy when they move and sleepy when they sit. It will also help if you give people something to occupy them when they can't relax.

- Display self-confidence at all times; don't let your worries show on your face. It will improve your subject's self-confidence, as well as build their confidence in you.

- If the bride and groom are in the same shoot, make sure the groom's body covers a part of the bride. It will make her look slimmer and the groom look stronger.

- Close-up shots reveal personality and make the viewer concentrate on the subject. Make your close-ups extreme. Crop out the left and right sides of the bride's face and construct your shot vertically. The result is a picture where the bride looks like a supermodel. Just don't forget to shoot at eye level or higher.

- Focus on the eyes when doing the close-ups. It has been said that the eyes are the mirror of the soul.

- Avoid shooting full-figured brides while being directly in front of them. Move around so your subject is at an angle. It will make the full-figured bride look slimmer and will add some interest to the picture.

- When standing on the left or right side of the bride, ask her to rotate her shoulders and head toward you while keeping the rest of her body stationary. It will make her bottom look smaller and will boost the picture's artistic qualities.

- Avoid placing a full-figured bride next to very tall, very skinny, or very small people. It will make her look awful.

- Avoid gaps between bodies, they add to body weight.

- If the bride is in a sitting position, angle your shot down from above her head and ask her to move her face toward the camera. It will tighten up the chin section of her face, which is a problem area for all full-figured women. The cheeks will benefit as well. And, of course, the double chins will also be gone.

- Capture emotions to make ordinary things look extraordinary. Happy faces, hugs, kisses, and greetings make the difference between a boring amateur shoot and a picture that looks like a piece of art.

RETOUCHING AND SPECIAL EFFECTS

Scan your negatives and retouch them on computer to get the most dramatic results and perfect color. This is very important because the general quality of the picture improves the look of the subjects. My tool of choice is Adobe Photoshop, but you can find a lot of alternative software if you can't afford this program. Just go to www.download.com and search for 'Image Editing.' Then upload your images to a website where you can order prints, like www.dotphoto.com, or make a CD and get your prints made at any pharmacy or professional photo lab.

- After you have scanned the pictures, make sure the color and contrast are right.

- Remove all the skin imperfections using the clone tool.

- Reduce the appearance of pores on your close-ups by blurring affected areas and adding some noise afterwards.

- Remove wrinkles using the clone tool if they unnecessarily age your bride.

- Kill 'Red Eye' by selecting and desaturating the affected areas.

- Crop the pictures properly if you didn't do it while shooting.

- Darken the shadows manually using the burn tool. It will help you make your bride look much leaner and hide the cheeks and the double chin.

- Create some lighting effects using levels, filters, and masking, if needed.

- Black and white or colorized pictures in most cases slim down your subject and add some drama to the shoot.

PHOTO TIPS

Cori Black of Cordi Photography in Detroit, Michigan, offers these tips:

- Couples: When shooting the bride and groom together (face to face), have them stand at a slight 45-degree angle from the camera, with part of the bride hidden by the groom.

- Standing: While the subjects are standing, avoid shooting side (body) shots 90-degrees in front of the camera.

- Sitting: Have the bride sit to the side of the groom leaning toward him, with one-third of her upper body behind his. Place her right hand on the groom's back and her left hand on the groom's mid-arm (left triceps); lean the bride's head towards the groom's shoulder.

- Gown: If plus-size brides choose to wear sleeveless gowns, I recommend that they drape a shawl or veil over their shoulders and upper arms for their photos. (Cameras see things differently than the human eye.)

- Posing alone: Have the bride stand with one foot slightly behind the other. Have her hold her bouquet mid-torso, in the mid-abdominal area. Again, make sure her shoulders and arms are draped with a shawl or veil if her gown is sleeveless.

- Lighting: Cori recommends shooting with continuous soft light (300 watts). The soft illumination helps smooth out full-figure curves.

Don't Let It End With The Party

There was a time in my life when I absolutely hated being in front of a mirror. I would often hide my body under oversized clothes and refuse to show any flesh at all, which was fine for the winter, but summertime was far less forgiving. Then one 98-degree day in July I had somewhere to go, and wearing long sleeves wasn't an option. So I reluctantly put on a sundress, prayed no one would look at me, and ventured out in public.

I had nearly completed my errands and thought I was home free when I heard someone call out, "Hey, sexy!" Of course I ignored the man since I was sure he was not—could not possibly—be talking to me. I looked around to see whom he was talking about and he pointed to me. I couldn't believe it. Up until that point I never fully realized the depth of my low self-esteem. I didn't feel worthy enough to receive a man's attention because I didn't love myself. I felt my love life as a "full-figured woman" read more like Stephen King than Danielle Steele. I lacked the pride of Maya Angelou's "Phenomenal Woman." I was at war with myself—and my self-esteem was the casualty. I had to make a decision: either I continued the war or I could call a truce and begin the healing process.

I called a truce. I took the time to get to love the woman I was, not some unreasonable, would-be facsimile. I started slowly by adding color to my otherwise "Darth Vader" wardrobe. Instead of finding things to hate in the mirror, I found things to like about my body. In time, like turned to love and my self-esteem made a miraculous recovery.

The amazing thing about this is once you love yourself, finding that special someone is easier. Far easier than you think. One day you meet him. He is warm, kind, gentle, loving, and sexy. He actually makes you feel good about yourself and loves everything about you. Your body becomes a work of art to be admired, not hidden. Every part of the body you have spent years calling "fat" or "too round" suddenly becomes "soft," "sexy," and "voluptuous."

I'm sure you know it's not easy for a full-figured woman to let herself love or be loved. Self-acceptance is a work in progress—old habits die a thousand deaths—but eventually they do die. Many a man has faced the challenge of dealing with our battle scars and lived to tell the tale.

I often look at the life of television star Delta Burke. When she was initially introduced to the public she had the body of a beauty queen, a fact not lost on any of the television shows in which she appeared. Then once she began to put on weight (before the eyes of the viewing public), her weight became fodder for late night talk show hosts and radio personalities. As a woman I could identify with her struggle, but it broke my heart to hear how merciless the jokes were. Still, despite her weight and in spite of her critics, she met and married Gerald McRaney in a service to rival any royal wedding. It was satisfying to see her walk out of the church with a man who loved her for who she was—a person and not just a "size."

DON'T LET IT END WITH THE PARTY

In 1996 I met a man with whom I spent nine years. Although we aren't together anymore the relationship helped me realize that I could be loved for who I am and not just some ideal. The lesson was a long time coming, but just like the commercial says, "I'm worth it."

The point is, you, like Delta, have found the man with whom you want to share your life. Be this your first and only wedding, or your second, third, or fourth trip down that wonderful path to marriage, this book is for you. I want to help you celebrate your love and your wedding; but most of all, I want you to use what you have learned, and celebrate yourself—every day of your life.

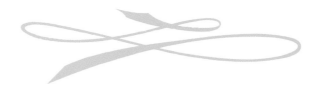

Author Biography

An epiphany happens in a moment— a sudden perception of essential nature or an intuitive grasp of reality. I've had two epiphanies in my life, moments when I suddenly understood so much more than I did even a moment before.

My youth was spent playing on Long Island, New York. My parents were Leonard Canton, Jr., a strong, compassionate man and a successful CPA, and Mary Wallace, a southern belle. From them I learned both the fiery independence for which New Yorkers are famous and the sweet charm and easy talk of the South. I grew up happy and strong in Black America.

At the tender age of four I discovered my life's passion—planning weddings. I had an Easy Bake oven, a tin box with a light bulb for heat, which I used to create wedding cakes. As I grew, my fascination turned to fashion and I purchased as many bridal magazines as I did *Teen Beat* and *Seventeen*. I was, and still am, a romantic. Eager for the Cinderella fantasy, I fell in love, and by age nineteen I was married. My husband and I were soon blessed with beautiful twin boys, and it seemed the fantasy would go on forever.

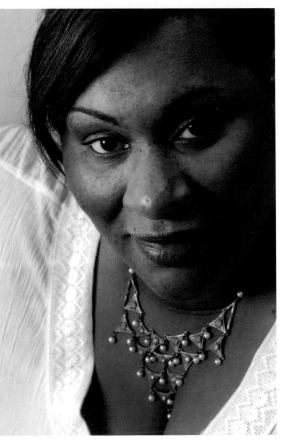

But the first of my life's epiphanies was just around the corner. The energy of youth soon gave way to the realities of life—my husband and I were unprepared for the responsibilities we had assumed. Our marriage ended in divorce and I found myself raising two young boys alone. I was twenty-three and quickly becoming an all too common statistic. With New York independence and the maturity that comes with epiphany, I resolved that my children would not suffer the usual difficulties of single-parent homes—but life wasn't done challenging me.

In the early 1990's I contracted uterine cancer. The disease was debilitating, both physically and emotionally. Wherever I went I carried an airsickness bag and frequently used it. Constant medical care left needle tracks in my arms. Imagine what people saw: a young, single Black mother, ill and exhausted, with tracks on her arms. I was the vision of an addict. If it had not been for my faith in the Divine, my love for my children, and the support I received from family and friends, I would have given in to the depression that was constantly nearby.

I can't overstate the value of a loving and supportive family.

My mother helped me enroll at Empire State College. My sister tended my boys, Sean and Scott, while I worked days and took classes at night. My father became the male role model for my sons, attending their school activities with us. He accompanied me to my endless medical treatments, taught me the fundamentals of business, and encouraged me to pursue my dream of becoming a wedding consultant. Without the energy of my family I wouldn't have had enough to succeed. But I did. In 1995, after countless treatments and what felt like a lifetime of indignity, I finally won my battle with cancer through one final treatment: a hysterectomy. I grieved the loss of future children, but I had long ago decided to never be a statistic.

Life was teaching me invaluable lessons in trust and self-confidence. The first was the result of my New York independence and my unpleasant divorce. This led to the decision to raise my children myself—an unpopular choice, to be sure, but I felt I'd lost too much control over my future and that of my children with the loss of trust in my husband. I had determined to see both my sons graduate from college, and I wanted nothing to interfere with that goal.

The second lesson came with the cancer and the loss of trust in my own body. It was a terrible feeling that I pray no one ever faces. Yet, nearly ten years of struggle had created strength within me that I didn't know I had. When I was finally free of the disease with my energy and dignity restored, I felt I could take on the whole world—so I did.

I helped plan several weddings that year, applying what I had learned from college and my parents. I wanted my own consulting business, and I finally had the strength and resources to do it. I chose to focus on the full-figured bride for two simple reasons: Genetics and ten years of trial had made me a full-figured woman, and I knew too many full-figured women who hadn't fully enjoyed their wedding day. The Southern charm I learned from my mother was ideal for working with the tender issue of self-image—but life still wasn't done challenging me.

Just as I started to build my reputation as a consultant I was struck down by another illness—Multiple Sclerosis. Cancer is a terrifying disease, but it's well known with several paths to a cure. Multiple Sclerosis, or MS, is much less known and doesn't yet have a cure. I fell into a state of denial. I attempted to live my life normally; I worked full-time and pursued my growing business on the weekends. As symptoms appeared, I ignored them. But the disease finally caught up with me in 1998.

In short, MS progressively attacks the nervous system until the victim is left disabled. Mild cases result in loss of muscle control, usually expressed as jerking limbs. Serious cases result in complete paralysis. Modern medicine combined with a healthy lifestyle can hold the disease at bay—but only if you're ready to deal with the issue. I was dead set on ignoring the whole thing, until a serious attack put me in a wheelchair. I was sure the disease and the world at large had won and I had lost. Then the second epiphany of my life happened.

I suddenly realized that I was no longer an inexperienced nineteen year-old. I was thirty-one years old. I had two wonderful sons showing all the promise of youth. I had a loving and supportive family and my faith in God, and I had a disease that I couldn't be rid of. But I also had the experience of having overcome another serious disease. All my life, I'd been fighting for control over my circumstances. Now I realized that I'd had that control all along. My life was my own, and I had others to live for. So, with the help of my family, I made the decision to get up out of the wheelchair.

Time would prove that my decision was much easier to make than to execute, but making it was half the battle. I focused my energy on getting back into the life I'd been building. Physical therapy and a healthy lifestyle soon lifted me from the wheelchair. It also fueled my desire to help full-figured women. The message I wanted to convey to them was suddenly clear—you need to be healthy and happy, whether you're a size two or 22! With the message clear in my mind, I worked hard to finish my college classes in business management. I also contacted my sons' school to apprise them of my situation and to monitor the boys' development. This, too, was therapeutic—a public admission of the changes in my life and a bold statement that I wasn't going to let those changes rule me.

One last therapy would change my life. To overcome my depression, I was encouraged to take up writing. I wrote and published two books: *You're Getting Married?* (Writers Club Press, 2000), the story of a plus-sized woman dealing with her upcoming wedding, and *Ms. Doesn't Stand for Multiple Sclerosis* (Writers Club Press, 2001), the story of a single parent dealing with MS. Both books are reflections of my own life and writing them helped me bring many of the emotions I had been feeling into the open. They also proved to me that I could communicate my passion for beautiful weddings to the world.

My re-energized passion for life was not lost on my sons. Unbeknownst to me they wrote an essay about my successes and submitted it to the Long Island chapter of the Multiple Sclerosis Society. Because of their efforts I received the MS Mother of the Year award for 2002. My pride in my sons redoubled—and redoubled again when they graduated in the top twenty percent of their class in 2005. Both have been accepted into college. One has been awarded the New York State Lottery's Leaders of Tomorrow Scholarship based on an essay about the true meaning of leadership, the result of his work with the National MS Society. My life's journey has been long and difficult, but I have won, and my family is proof of it.

But this isn't the end of my story. Graduating from college, raising two sons, building a successful consulting business, writing my books, and working with my publishers convinced me that I could help women like myself with more than their wedding day—I can help them through their writing. I am now the managing partner of a small literary agency, the Canton Smith Agency, that's dedicated to first-time women authors. Our goal is to represent literary artistry in a commercial venue without sacrificing artistic integrity. This isn't always easy. Authors often see their work as art, but publishers must see it as a commodity. Still, it can be done. We currently have twenty-eight clients, seven of whom have signed publishing contracts.

The challenges of life could have torn me down and made me one of the statistics I feared so much, but the strength of my faith and family buoyed me up. It made me so much more than I ever thought I could be. We are now three generations looking forward to a fourth, and life couldn't be sweeter.

Chamein

Appendix: Makeup

Skin Preparation

Eye Cream

A good eye cream or gel for day wear will help to reduce puffiness and provide a better surface for the application of your concealer. There are a lot of wonderful eye creams to be found in department stores: Lancome, Clarins, Clinique, Estée Lauder, and Prescriptives to name a few. However, your local drugstore has a large selection of eye creams which not only work well, but don't empty your pocketbook. Oil of Olay, Ponds, L'Oréal, and Revlon are all available nationally.

Moisturizer

This is the most essential step of your makeup routine, even if you have oily skin. A well-moisturized face produces less oil, allowing your makeup to stay in place longer. Unless you have extremely dry skin, use an oil free moisturizer. (Try Kiehls or Neutrogena.)

Primer

Apply this after your moisturizer, wait five minutes, then apply your foundation. Most primers have a silicone base which will provide a smooth, even surface for foundation. Primer is especially helpful for those with large pores, acne scars, or age lines, as it can fill in those areas. Primers are great but they aren't miracle products, so don't expect them to erase every imperfection. (Try Laura Mercier or English Ideas.)

Concealer

Apply after primer and before or after foundation (the choice is yours). Concealers are a thicker formulation than foundation because they are meant to provide more coverage and staying power on small areas. Use a light touch around your eyes if you have age lines as concealer can accentuate them. Based on the type of foundation you use, you may not need a separate concealer, so read the information on foundation products before purchasing one. (Try Kevyn Aucoin, Surreal Skin, Lancôme, Estée Lauder, Fashion Fair, Iman, Sephora, Revlon, Maybelline, Neutrogena, Almay, or Max Factor.)

Foundation

Tinted Moisturizer

Provides very sheer coverage. This is not a good product for brides, since even those with good skin usually require more coverage when they are having pictures taken. Additionally, brides using sunscreen at an outdoor wedding need to know that almost all sunscreens contain large amounts of Titanium Dioxide, which will give their skin a whitish cast in pictures. (Try Bobbi Brown or Paula Dorf.)

Liquid Foundation

This is the most popular type of foundation. It is fairly thin, but in conjunction with concealer, it can provide a medium amount of coverage. Liquid is best for people with good skin. Liquid foundations are not recommended for those with very oily skin since liquid formulas slide easily. It is also best to avoid liquid formulations if you have acne scarring or large pores because the foundation will sink into them but not fill them, making them more obvious. (Try Armani or MAC.)

Cream Foundation

Thicker than liquid but thinner than a stick foundation, cream foundations offer great coverage without looking heavy. It is possible to skip using a concealer if you wear a cream foundation since creams can be thick enough to conceal. If you find cream a bit too heavy, use moisturizer to thin it out. Cream foundations are not the best choice for women with age lines, since it may accentuate them. (Try Shu Uemura Nobara or William Tuttle.)

Stick Foundation

This is the heaviest coverage foundation. It is the best option if you have a lot of acne or major pigment differentiation on your face. It is important to use a light touch and blend well, or it will look thick and mask-like. Like a cream foundation, you can forgo a separate concealer if you use a stick foundation. (Try Bobbi Brown or Smashbox.)

Blush

Cream or Gel

This type of blush is great if you want to create a soft glow. Do not use this product on cheekbones, since it may look streaky. It is best rubbed gently into the apples of the cheeks for a sweet, blushing look. Be careful with these products. They are messy to apply, dry very fast, and can stain your hands. (Try Benefit.)

APPENDIX: MAKEUP

Powder

This is the most popular form of blush and the one most often recommended. It should be applied with a big round brush for a soft look, or with a large angled brush to define your cheekbones. Choose a soft shade of blush such as a peach, soft pink, or cinnamon color for the apples of your cheeks, and a darker color for contour. (Try Paula Dorf or MAC.)

Eyebrows

Brow Gel

Brow gel will make unruly eyebrows lie flat.

Eyebrow Pencil or Wax

Use an eyebrow pencil to lightly trace the shape of your eyebrows to determine their natural arch. If brows are sparse, carefully pencil in the brow, using short, blending strokes. Match the color of the pencil to your natural hair color. Don't let the brow get too dark. You can also use the pencil to fill in thinner spots on heavier eyebrows, matching the color of your brows. (Prior to doing your makeup, if brows are full and bushy, use the penciled outline to define the area you want to pluck or wax. This will prevent over-plucking and over-waxing.)

Eye Shadow

Powder

The most common type of shadow by far. For your wedding eye makeup, use powder shadows exclusively; they are the least messy and longest lasting. Avoid using a powder with too much sparkle since it might drop down onto your face during the course of the day. (Try MAC or Bobbi Brown.)

Cream

This type of shadow is not recommended for wedding makeup. Creams tend to smudge, crease, and transfer to unwanted places. The only exception would be a cream to powder formula, which goes on as a cream but dries to a powder. The only place to use an actual cream shadow on your wedding day would be under your brow bone as a highlight. (Try Urban Decay or MAC Paints.)

Eyeliner

Pencil

This is the most commonly used liner. To avoid a harsh line, sharpen the pencil and then soften it slightly by rubbing it on your finger. Avoid putting this beneath your lower lashes if you think you might cry. (Try Paula Dorf or Prestige.)

Liquid

This type of liner is intimidating to many people. It requires a steady hand, but the brush and the formulation do make for a very smooth application. Don't use this type if you've never tried it before. And definitely choose a waterproof formula. (Try Lancôme.)

Powder

This is a good choice for people who are nervous about having a steady hand because it's very easy to blend. You can buy a powder made specifically to use as eyeliner, or just use one of your dark eye shadows. Use a straight liner brush with powder liner. (Try MAC or Benefit.)

Eyelashes

False Lashes

There are two basic types—strips and individual lashes. Strip eyelashes are not a good idea for your wedding because they look fake. Individual eyelashes are actually about three lashes grouped together. They create a subtly dramatic look, but they can be difficult to apply. You will need to have a steady hand, good placement technique, and an eye for symmetry to make them the same on both eyes.

Eyelash Glue

Essential if you are using false lashes. Choose either the clear or black glue because the white glue doesn't dry completely clear. (Try Duo or Ricky's Brand.)

Tweezers

In addition to getting rid of spare hairs (though you should have waxed or tweezed your brows a few days before for the perfect look!), this is what you will need to use to apply your false lashes. (Try Tweezerman.)

Eyelash Curler

Don't be afraid! This is a quick and painless way to amplify your lashes. Make sure you get all your eyelashes in it before clamping down, then "walk" it away from your eye until you have released your lashes. Your eyes will look twice as big. (Try Kevyn Aucoin or Shu Uemura.)

Clear Mascara

Use clear mascara to lengthen your lashes without adding color when you don't need it. Makes the eyes pop and keeps the black smudges off your face, especially if you get emotional during your wedding.

Mascara

Mascara makes a huge difference in the look of your lashes. It can also make a huge mess if it runs on your face, so find a waterproof formula. If you have very pale lashes, you don't need to wear a black; a brown or black/brown is fine. Make sure you comb the lashes through after you apply the mascara to avoid lumpiness. (Try Maybelline Great Lash, Estée Lauder, or English Ideas.)

Powder

Loose Powder

This type of powder is packaged with a shaker top. The advantage of loose powder is its soft, matte coverage. The disadvantage is that it can be messy, especially for touch-ups, so try a translucent or colorless version. If you are darker skinned, look for a translucent powder with a yellowish tone. (Try Urban Decay Universal Powder, or Ben Nye Banana Powder.)

Pressed Powder

This type of powder comes in a compact. It should basically match your foundation color. Pressed powder offers good coverage and is recommended if you are wearing tinted moisturizer or liquid foundation. (Try Christian Dior.)

Lips

Lip Primer

If you have very dry lips, this will soften them and allow your lipstick and liner to go on more easily. If you are a bit older, choose an anti-aging primer; it has ingredients that fill in the lines around your lips to prevent your lipstick from bleeding. (Try English Ideas.)

Lip Liner

Choose a shade very close to your natural lip color. Sharpen the pencil and then slightly dull the edge on your finger. Apply to the entire surface of your lips to create a long lasting base for your lipstick. (Try MAC or Bobbi Brown.)

Lipstick

Choose a fairly natural shade with some warmth to it. Apply to your lips, blot, and then reapply. (Try Bobbi Brown or MAC.)

Lip Sealant

Apply this after the lipstick and before the gloss. It will help keep your lipstick color on, but may make your lips look dry. Use a touch of gloss after applying to counteract dryness. (Try English Ideas.)

Lip Gloss

A little lip gloss goes a long way. Gloss can make your lips appear fuller and more sensual. Skip the gloss or use it sparingly if you are over 40. (Try Lancôme Juicy Tubes or Urban Decay XXX Shine.)

Finishing

Fixative

This is a product usually only sold at professional makeup stores. It's a spray that you apply to your face after you have applied all your makeup to help keep your makeup in place. It really works, but it will make your makeup harder to take off at the end of the night! (Try Kryolan or Ben Nye Final Seal.)

Glossary

Clothing design and attribute terms vary greatly due to ever changing market trends and local culture. However, this glossary adheres to traditional wedding gown definitions.

Many terms in this glossary are not discussed elsewhere in the book due to their being parochial, esoteric, redundant, or obsolete. They are often misused in the wedding industry and should be avoided.

A-Line Silhouette

The A-line silhouette is the most common silhouette. It has a formfitting bodice that (usually) flows seamlessly to a full skirt that flares from the waist. (See A-Line Skirt.) Generally works well on all body types, and the construction of the gown is such that it easily lends itself to all body shapes.

A-Line Skirt

A skirt that is fitted at the waist and flares out in an A-line shape toward the hem. (See A-Line Silhouette.)

Angel Veil

A veil cut wide at the sides like angel wings.

Antebellum Waist

A dropped form of the basque waist; most often created using the curved basque waist. The result is an old-fashioned look reminiscent of the southern belles of the mid-1800s.

Apron

An overskirt that creates a layered effect across the front of the skirt and closes at the waist, either at the back or the side of the skirt. (An apron-style overskirt that closes at the front of the waist is called a redingote or redingcote).

Asymmetric Neckline

A compound neckline created by mixing combinations of sleeve, strap, neckline, or bodice on the right and left sides of the gown. For example, a single-shoulder tank top neckline would be an asymmetrical neckline. Many necklines can be modified to be asymmetric.

Asymmetric Waist

A waist design that creates asymmetry, either by applied design or through the lay of the cloth.

Back Drape

A length of material that is attached either at the shoulder or at the waist and flows down the back to the floor. In some cases, it can be removed.

Back Neckline

The neckline on the back of the bodice. Most necklines can be used and need not be the same as the front neckline.

Back Veil

A veil attached at some point on the back of the head that falls straight down the back rather than covering the sides of the head. Usually used with updo hair styles.

Backline or Back Line

(See Back Neckline.)

Backpiece

A headpiece that is worn on the back of the head.

Ball Silhouette

Sometimes called the traditional silhouette. It is characterized by a very full skirt that is fitted at the waist and flares to a formal length. The skirt waist is seamed at the natural waistline and can be of various styles. It suits all body shapes and is especially good for rectangle and pear shapes.

Ballerina Neckline

A compound neckline created by combining a scoop, square, or sweetheart neckline with spaghetti straps.

Balloon Sleeve

(See Bishop Sleeve.)

Band Collar Neckline

(See Wedding Band or High Collar Neckline.)

Basque Waist

This waist starts at or just below the natural waistline and dips in the front creating a "V" shape. It features a fitted bodice. This type of waist generally works well on most body shapes. (A curved basque waist comes to a "U" instead of a "V.")

Bateau Neckline

A high, wide neckline that often follows just be-

low the line of the collarbone and runs across the front and back, meeting at the shoulders. It is the same depth in front as it is in back.

Bell Sleeve

This sleeve is gathered over the armhole and flares at the hem. It is a version of the cape sleeve.

Birdcage Veil

A blusher attached to a hat.

Bishop Sleeve

A full sleeve similar to the Juliet sleeve, with the pouf extending down the arm and gathered in at the elbow or the wrist.

Blouson Bodice

A non-form-shaping (non-corseted) bodice made only of fabric. The traditional blouson bodice has a drooping fullness in its fabric from shoulder to waist that is gathered at or below the waist.

Blusher

A piece of veil illusion used to cover the face. Varies from chin-length to elbow-length.

Boat Neckline

(See Bateau Neckline.)

Bodice

(1) The upper part of a woman's dress, including straps and waist. (See Compound Neckline and Empire Silhouette.)

(2) That part of the upper gown that covers the midsection, but does not include the neckline,

waist, or straps. There are three midsection bodice styles: corseted, fitted, and blouson.

Bolero

A bolero is a loose jacket or coat that is open at the front. Bolero jackets can be fingertip length, waist length, or shorter. The duster-like coat version is usually three-quarter or floor length.

Boned Bodice

(See Corseted Bodice.)

Boning

The tensioned material that creates the distinctive shape of a corset. Boning was originally made of whale bone. Modern boning can be almost anything, including elastic nylon, shaped leather, fiberglass, or wood.

Bouffant Skirt

A sheer, puffed-out skirt often made of stiffened silk, tulle, rayon, or nylon net. Bouffant skirts are often very full (see Ball Silhouette), and accompanied by a hoop slip.

Bow

A large bow tied at the back of the waist or elsewhere on the gown.

Box Pleated Skirt

Features a natural waist with deep pleats of parallel fabric folds.

Brocade

A rich silk fabric with raised patterns in gold and silver; a fabric characterized by raised designs.

Elastic threads can be added to create stretch brocade.

Bun Ring

A type of crown headpiece. A bun ring is worn around a bun in the bride's hair.

Bustle

A gather of cloth at the back of the waist. A bustle is often created by "gathering up" the train to prevent it from dragging along the floor, grass, or other surfaces where it may get soiled. Bustles can be positioned over the skirt or under the skirt. There are three basic types of bustles:

Traditional Bustle: The train is pulled up to the back of the waist and held in place by either hooks, snaps, or buttons that have been placed in a straight line across the back so that the bustle will look even. The bottom of the skirt should be straight after the bustle is fastened. This bustle works well if there is not a lot of decoration on the train and the decoration falls closer to the hemline.

French (or Victorian) Bustle: Ribbons are attached at the underside of the gown or to the inner slip. The two ends of the ribbons are tied together at each bustle point to draw the excess fabric of the train under the skirt. It works well for trains that have a lot of detail and lace around the edge.

Pickup Bustle: This is used on dresses that are not elaborate. The excess fabric of the train is drawn up and attached at the midpoint of the skirt to a discrete hook or button. (Midpoint is usually a little lower than the small of a woman's back.) (See Train.)

Butterfly Cuff

A poet cuff that is elongated away from the bottom of the wrist and possibly cut or split along the wrist. (See Butterfly Sleeve.)

Butterfly Sleeve

The butterfly sleeve is a modified renaissance sleeve that has been split along the arm from the elbow to the cuff, giving the impression of butterfly wings.

Butterfly Veil

A veil that is oval-shaped and folded in half. Ribbon edging follows a crescent shape rather than a straight line.

Button Hook

A slender, long-handled hook similar to a crochet needle that is used to close the buttons on long gloves. The hook is passed through the buttonhole and used to grasp the button, which is then pulled back through the buttonhole.

Cap

A brimless headpiece covering some or all of the crown of the head.

Cape Sleeve

This sleeve fits smoothly over the armhole and flares out from the shoulder, giving the appearance of a cape. A gathered form of the cape sleeve is known as a bell sleeve.

Capelet Train

(See Watteau Train.)

Cascade Train

(See Tiered Skirt.)

Cascade Veil

A veil having two or more tiers or layers of veil illusion.

Chiffon

A sheer fabric, especially of silk.

Choker Neckline

(See Wedding Band Neckline.)

Classic Bridal Look

Involves the overall look of bridal fashions. Characterized by simple, tailored lines. (See Traditional Bridal Look and Modern Bridal Look.)

Coat Glove

(See Three-Quarter Glove.)

Column Silhouette

Also known as the straight silhouette. This is a sheath silhouette that forms a straight line from shoulder to ankle but is not formfitting below the hips. (See also Sheath Silhouette.) The column's construction is rather unforgiving of any figure flaws. An hourglass shape is best suited for this gown.

Column Skirt

Straight-line skirt with no flare or fullness at the waistline or hem. (See Column Silhouette.)

GLOSSARY

Comb Headpiece

A plain or decorated hair comb used to hold a veil in place.

Compound Neckline

A compound neckline is any combination of sleeves, straps, neckline, or bodice that creates a unique appearance. Common compound necklines are asymmetric, ballerina, contessa, halter, off-the-shoulder, and strapless.

Contessa Neckline

A compound neckline created with dropped sleeves and a strapless bodice. This neckline is characterized by the top line of the dropped sleeves and the neckline forming a line across the body.

Contessa Sleeves

Generally a dropped, short, often puffed sleeve attached to a strapless bodice or held in place with elastic. (See Dropped Sleeve, Sleeve Length, and Melon Sleeve.)

Coronet

(See Tiara Headpiece.)

Corseted Bodice

A formfitting bodice that incorporates either boning or other tensioned material to hold the bodice in place. It is often constructed with a laced closure, a zipper, or a snap closure. It is styled after the fashion of ladies' undergarments by the same name. Corseted bodices can be used with most necklines and waist styles.

Crown Headpiece

A headpiece worn on the crown of the head either with or without a veil. Unlike tiaras, crowns are usually a uniform width circling the head.

Cuff

The hem of a sleeve or glove that encircles the wrist or arm. A cuff may or may not incorporate a band. Different types are butterfly, fitted, poet, pointed, scalloped, and straight. Straight, scalloped, and fitted cuffs can be narrow or wide.

Curved Basque Waist

A modified basque or antebellum waist that comes to a curved "U" rather than a pointed "V." (See Antebellum Waist and Basque Waist.)

Décolletage Neckline

Considered a neckline attribute, any cleavage-revealing, plunging neckline.

Diamond Neckline

(See Keyhole Neckline.)

Dolman Sleeve

This is a loose sleeve that is normally cut as an extension of the bodice and designed without a socket for the shoulder. It creates a deep, wide armhole that starts at or slightly above the waist and narrows to a point on the arm or wrist, depending on length.

Dropped Shoulders

Characterized by the shoulder/sleeve seam falling below the shoulder.

Dropped Waist

A waistline that falls below the body's natural waistline.

Elbow Glove

This glove is measured from the tip of the middle finger to a point one to three inches above the elbow. It is generally a 10- to 14-button glove.

Empire Bodice

A bodice that ends just below the bustline. (See Empire Waist.)

Empire Silhouette

A column silhouette making use of an empire waist. (See Empire Waist.) This silhouette is reminiscent of the gowns worn in the movie Emma. It features a narrow bodice complimented with any neckline style and gathered or sewn high at the waist (just beneath the bustline) to a slender and graceful skirt. An empire silhouette works well on pear shapes and thick waists.

Empire Waist

This waistline lies just below the bust. Traditionally, the skirt below is a column skirt. (See Empire Bodice and Empire Silhouette.)

Fichu Neckline

Considered a neckline attribute, fabric is wrapped around the shoulders and tucked into the bodice to look like an attached shawl.

Fingerless Gloves

Traditionally, gloves completely enclose the fingers. However, modern designs allow parts of the fingers and hands to be exposed. Fingerless gloves allow brides to combine the elegance of a long pointed sleeve and the convenience of not wearing a glove during their ceremony with the sophistication of a glove.

Half-Finger: Fingers and thumb are exposed from the first knuckle to the finger tip.

Fingerless: A glove of any length cut with a square end over the knuckles of the hand.

Mitt: A fingerless glove of any length with an index-finger or middle-finger loop that draws the glove to a point over the back of the hand. The mitt is sometimes erroneously called a gauntlet.

Fishtail Train

Unlike traditional trains (which are gathered in at the waist), fishtail trains are fitted at the waist and flare from the knees into a short train.

Fit-and-Flare Silhouette

(See Mermaid Silhouette.)

Fitted Bodice

A formfitting bodice where the shape is created by the cut of the cloth. It is never strapless.

Fitted Cuff

A cuff that fits snugly around the wrist or arm. Pointed and straight cuffs are fitted cuffs. Poet and butterfly cuffs are not.

Fitted Sleeve

Any length sleeve that is cut to fit the arm from shoulder to cuff. Fitted sleeves on wedding gowns are usually long and may include a pointed cuff at the wrist.

Flare Skirt

(See A-Line Skirt.)

Flounce

A wide piece of fabric or lace (often gathered) that is attached at the hem of a skirt.

Fluted Skirt

A gathered skirt that produces vertical grooves when hanging straight.

Flyaway Veil

A stiff, shoulder-length cascade veil that flares dramatically.

Fountain Veil

A veil normally made with tulle or illusion netting that is gathered at the crown of the head to create a cascade effect around the face.

Frontline or Front Neckline

The neckline used on the front of the bodice. (See Neckline.)

Gauntlet Glove

Any glove with an equestrian-style or flared opening. Usually only the longer gloves (8-button and larger) will be of this style. They are appropriate for wear with most sleeve lengths. The arm pieces of gauntlets are customarily worn over the sleeve of your blouse, gown, or coat. (Though improper, the opera mitt is often called a gauntlet.)

Georgette

A sheer crepe fabric woven from hard-twisted yarns to produce a dull pebbly surface.

Gigot Sleeve

Loose and full from shoulder to just below the elbow, then shaped to the arm, often ending in a point. (Also called a leg-of-mutton sleeve.)

Glove

A covering for the hand having separate sections for each of the fingers and the thumb, and often extending part way up the arm.

Glove Lengths

The length of a glove is traditionally expressed in "buttons," an antique French unit of measure which is slightly longer than one inch. Button measures are customarily taken from the bottom of the thumb seam to the top of the glove, and the actual length of the glove is six to seven inches longer than the length in buttons. Modern glove makers still occasionally use the button unit of measure, although most are standardizing on fixed measurements in inches starting at the tip of the middle finger.

0–2 button: Also known as short, shorties, and wrist gloves. These are generally six to nine inches long and will fall just below, at, or just above the wrist. These gloves are easily removed during the wedding ceremony and held by a bridesmaid.

4-button: These gloves are 10 to 11 inches long and cover the wrist, reaching a couple of inches up onto the forearm.

6-button: Twelve to thirteen inches long, these

gloves reach well up onto the forearm. Many gauntlet gloves are this length. The six- and eight-button lengths are known as three-quarter gloves, and sometimes as coat gloves.

8-button: Fourteen to fifteen inches long, this type of glove reaches to the upper forearm. This is also known as a three-quarter glove, and is the style worn by Audrey Hepburn in Breakfast at Tiffany's.

12-button: Approximately 18 to 19 inches long, this type of glove reaches up to or just over the wearer's elbow. Also known as an elbow glove. Many have mousquetaire wrist openings, but they should not be confused with the 16-button glove.

16-button: Twenty-two to twenty-three inches long. This is the classic opera glove and as a general rule, comes with a mousquetaire wrist opening.

21-button: Twenty-seven to twenty-nine inches long, this glove generally reaches all the way to the wearer's armpits. This is possibly the most dramatic length of glove and is generally worn only with strapless or sleeveless evening outfits.

Halo Headpiece

A circlet of any type circling the head, either resting on the crown of the head or placed low on the forehead. Common halo headpieces are wreaths and V-bands.

Halter Neckline

A compound neckline created by combining a sleeveless bodice and a scoop, square, or V-neck neckline with any halter other than spaghetti straps (traditionally a neck halter).

Halter Straps

Generally, any over-the-shoulder strapped and sleeveless neckline that does not use spaghetti straps. Halter straps come in three styles:

Straight Halters: A strap flowing up and over the shoulder. (Spaghetti straps are almost always a straight halter style.)

Cross Halters: A strap flowing over the shoulder and across the back to the other shoulder, the two straps crossing in the back, or the reverse where the straps cross over the breasts and then flow straight down behind each shoulder.

Neck Halters: A single strap that flows up from one side of the bodice, around the back of the neck, and down the other side of the bodice.

Hanging Sleeve

A sleeve of any length that does not cover the shoulders. Most commonly a very short sleeve (almost a strap) that hangs gently off the shoulders. Off-the-shoulder gowns are strapless gowns with hanging sleeves.

Hat

A headpiece that partially or completely covers the crown of the head. Hats can combine both veils and blushers. Hats without brims are known as caps.

Headband

A band that runs over the top of the head from ear to ear to hold a veil in place.

GLOSSARY

Headpiece

An object worn on the head both for decoration and to attach the veil. The following are common headpieces: backpiece, bun ring, cap, comb, crown, halo, hat, headband, spray, and tiara. The V-band and wreath headpieces are popular types of the halo headpiece.

Hemline

Tradition has given names to hemlines (skirt lengths). No specific length defines any given name as they are often measured to various points on the bride's body. Common hemline names are:

Mini: Measured to a point above the knees.

Street: Measured to a point just below the knees.

Intermission: Measured to a point midway between the knees and ankles. (Also known as tea length or midi length.)

Ballet: Measured to the ankles. (Also known as ankle length or ballerina length.)

Floor: The skirt lightly touches the floor on all sides.

Hi-Lo: The hem is higher in the front than in the back. The most common configuration is an intermission hem in front and a floor hem in back.

High Collar Neckline

(See Wedding Band Neckline.)

Hoop Slip

A slip constructed with stiff tensioned hoops (similar to the material used in corsets) to create the ball silhouette's full skirt shape. Reminiscent of the full skirts worn by Southern women in the mid- to late-1800s.

Illusion

This is a sheer material such as a fine tulle that is used for veils and accents on gowns and skirts. It produces a soft, illusory look.

Illusion Bodice

A bodice or yoke made of sheer material and added to other necklines to give the illusion of a second neckline. Tends to grant the benefits of both necklines to the wearer. For example, a sweetheart neckline to emphasize the bosom combined with a jewel illusion neckline to lengthen perceived height.

Illusion Glove

Any glove made out of a sheer material.

Illusion High Neckline

A specific illusion bodice created by combining a scoop, square, or sweetheart neckline with a wedding band illusion neckline. (See Wedding Band Neckline.)

Illusion Skirt

An overskirt made of illusion. (See Overskirt.)

Illusion Sleeve

A sleeve made from sheer material, such as tulle.

Inverted-V Waist

A waistline, usually raised, that forms an inverted-V in front.

Jacquard

A fabric of intricate, variegated weave or pattern.

Jewel Neckline

A round neckline that follows the base of the neck.

Juliet Cap

A cap that snugly fits the crown of the head and is ornately encrusted with pearls and sequins.

Juliet Sleeve

A long fitted sleeve with a small pouf at the shoulder.

Keyhole Neckline

A neckline attribute with an opening just below the neckline on the front or back of a garment. The opening can be cut in different shapes (e.g., keyhole, diamond, oval, teardrop, etc.).

Leg-of-Mutton Sleeve

(See Gigot Sleeve.)

Linen

Cloth woven from thread made of flax.

Low Waist

(See Dropped Waist.)

Lycra

A spandex, synthetic fiber.

Madonna Veil

(See Birdcage Veil.)

Mandarin Collar

A wedding band neckline with a notched-V in front.

Mantilla

A veil that features lace-trimmed netting (with or without a simple base) that is draped over the head. The mantilla gently frames the face and is often secured with an elegant comb. This Spanish-inspired veil was made popular by Jacqueline (Jackie) Lee Bouvier when she married John Kennedy.

Melon Sleeve

A large puff covering the shoulder to a point above the elbow, leaving the forearm bare.

Mermaid Silhouette

This silhouette hugs the body until it reaches the knees or just above, and then ends in a dramatic flare. This silhouette makes use of the trumpet skirt. The body-hugging gown can be designed with or without a waistline. It looks best on an hourglass shape, but with a waistline, is usable by rectangle shapes as well.

Mesh

A woven, knit, or knotted material of open texture with evenly spaced holes.

GLOSSARY

Mitt

(See Fingerless Glove.)

Modern Bridal Look

Usually used in reference to gowns with a dramatic fit or design. (See also Traditional Bridal Look and Classic Bridal Look.)

Modesty Panels

Detachable pieces of cloth designed to cover the arms, back, and/or chest of a dress that normally has a low neckline or no sleeves.

Mousquetaire Buttons

The name descends from the buttons on gloves worn by the French Musketeers (Mousquetaires). They consist of one or more buttons at the wrist of 12-button and longer gloves to assist in their removal. When closed, the glove fits snug at the wrist. When open, the glove is loose and easy to remove. Mousquetaire buttons are often used on the backs of baseball gloves.

Muslin

A plain-woven, sheer to coarse cotton fabric.

Narrow Cuff

A fitted cuff incorporating a narrow band. Dolman sleeves frequently use narrow cuffs.

Natural Waist

(1) The indentation between the hips and the rib cage.

(2) A seam or waistband that falls at the natural curve of the body.

Neckline

The line of the neck opening of a garment. (See the definitions of individual necklines for their descriptions.) The basic necklines are scoop, square, sweetheart, V-neck, wedding band, jewel, and bateau. Other common neckline names include asymmetric, décolletage, keyhole, portrait, Queen Anne, Queen Elizabeth, and tank top. These and still other neckline names refer to combinations of necklines, bodices, and straps which are common in the wedding industry.

Neckline Attribute

Any of a number of design attributes that can be applied to a neckline. Most attributes are decorative in nature, though some can significantly modify how you are perceived by other people. Neckline attributes include décolletage, notched-V, keyhole, scalloped, portrait, and fichu.

Neckline Decoration

A modification to a neckline that is used to decorate or enhance the bustline. Neckline decorations include scalloping, collaring, and a notched-V.

Notched-V

A neckline attribute; a V-shaped cut over the chest on any neckline. The notched-V decoration is most often used with the square neckline. A décolletage neckline is often created by combining a notched-V decoration with a sweetheart neckline. A notched-V in a plain, high collar neckline is commonly called a mandarin collar.

Off-the-Shoulder Neckline

A compound neckline created by combining any strapless neckline with a hanging sleeve. (See also

Contessa Sleeves, Hanging Sleeves, and Strapless Bodice.)

Opera Glove

Any 16-button and longer glove length. The traditional opera glove is the 16-button length, and measures from the tip of the middle finger to a point approximately four inches above the elbow. Many manufacturers refer to any of their longer gloves as opera gloves.

Opera Mitt

A 16-button length Mitt that is often (and incorrectly) described as a gauntlet. (See Fingerless Glove.)

Organdy

A very fine transparent muslin with a stiff finish.

Organza

A sheer dress fabric (as of silk or nylon) resembling organdy.

Overskirt

One skirt lying on top of another. Illusion overskirts are often used with the column silhouette. Aprons and redingotes are specific styles of overskirts.

Pannier

Gathered fabric worn on the hips over the sides of the skirt for an effect of fullness.

Peplum

A short section of cloth attached to the back of the skirt. Often layered to create a cascade effect leading to the train. Also a flounce attached at the waistline of a dress or blouse that fastens in the front.

Pickup Skirt

A design element on a skirt where the fabric is picked up at various points and attached to the skirt. It creates a full, voluminous look.

Picture Hat

Features a very large brim often elaborately decorated with laces, beads, and sequins.

Plain Waist

A waistline that is formed by the cut of the gown and is otherwise unadorned.

Poet Cuff

Flares from the wrist, usually uniformly, to cover the back of the hand. (See Poet Sleeve.)

Poet Sleeve

A poet sleeve is fitted at the top and flares from the elbow to the wrist. It can be gathered into a cuff.

Pointed Cuff

A cuff that incorporates a point over the back of the hand.

Portrait Neckline

(1) The traditional portrait neckline is created by combining a scoop neckline with a collar.

(2) A shawl-like collar that wraps the shoulders.

GLOSSARY

Pouf

(1) A bouffant or fluffy feature on any garment or accessory.

(2) A bouffant or gathering of veil illusion at the crown of the head.

Princess Silhouette

Though traditionally there are differences between the A-line and princess silhouettes, time is rapidly merging the two into a single silhouette. Most A-line and princess silhouettes seen in today's catalogs are indistinguishable from each other. Traditionally, the princess silhouette is a slim-fitting gown with a gently flared skirt and vertical seams flowing from the shoulders to the hem. It is flattering to most shapes but unlike the A-line, there are exceptions. If you have a thick waist or are pear-shaped, the princess line will draw attention to flaws you would rather conceal.

Puffed (Poufed) Sleeve

Any sleeve that incorporates a pouf. (See also the Gigot Sleeve, Juliet Sleeve, and Melon Sleeve.)

Queen Anne Neckline

This neckline combines a wedding band collar (open in front) and a scoop, square, or (traditionally) sweetheart neckline. It cups the back of the neck in a choker effect, then sculpts low across the chest to create a low neckline. (See the Wedding Band Neckline.)

Queen Elizabeth Neckline

This is a very high neckline, open in front and flared in back. It slopes gently and becomes narrower as it circles the neck to the front, ending in a V-neck, square, or sweetheart neckline. (See the Wedding Band Neckline.)

Raised Waist

A waistline that is above the natural waist but below the bosom. (See Empire Waist.)

Rayon

Any of a group of smooth textile fibers made from regenerated cellulose extruded through minute holes; a rayon yarn, thread, or fabric.

Redingote/Redingcote

(1) A fitted outer garment: as a dress with a front gore of contrasting material.

(2) An overskirt that closes in front at the waist and opens down the length of the skirt to reveal the underskirt. The reverse of an apron.

(3) A woman's lightweight coat open at the front.

Renaissance Sleeve

A long sleeve that is loosely fitted from shoulder to elbow then widens dramatically from elbow to wrist, leaving the wrist free.

Ring Finger Opening

A slit in the ring finger of a glove that allows the bride to expose her finger during the ring ceremony without first removing her gloves.

Round Neckline

(See Jewel Neckline and Scoop Neckline.)

Sabrina Neckline

A version of the bateau neckline. It runs slightly higher than the bateau neckline, along (rather than below) the collarbone.

Satin

Fabric (as of silk) in satin weave with lustrous face and dull back.

Scalloped Cuff

A cuff that has had a scalloped effect applied to it.

Scalloped Neckline

Any neckline that has had a scalloped effect applied to it. (See Neckline Attribute.)

Scalloped Hem

A hemline that has had a scalloped effect applied to it.

Scoop Neckline

A low, U-shaped or round neckline. On a sleeveless gown, it is known as a tank top neckline.

Sheath Silhouette

Sheath silhouettes have a formfitting bodice and a straight or close-fitting skirt. The skirt is often ankle length and sometimes has a slit in either the front, side, or back to make walking easier. Gowns of this silhouette often have detachable trains. It is a slim, body-hugging gown with a seamless waistline. As with the mermaid silhouette, this gown works best on hourglass shapes.

Shirred Waist

Fabric is gathered to make a horizontal panel at the waist.

Short Glove

(See Wrist Glove.)

Shortie Glove

(See Wrist Glove.)

Silhouette

The outline or general shape of a wedding gown. The basic gown silhouettes are A-line, ball, column, empire, mermaid, and sheath.

Silk

A fine continuous protein fiber produced by various insect larvae usually for cocoons. Especially, a lustrous tough elastic fiber produced by silkworms and used for textiles.

Skirt

The part of a wedding gown that covers the body from the waist down. Skirts come in various styles: bouffant, box pleated, empire, gathered, hi-lo (see Hemline), pickup, tiered, A-line, and trumpet. Design elements that can be applied to the skirt are aprons, flounces, back drapes, an overskirt, a bustle, a pannier, a redingote (or redingcote), and a peplum.

Skirt Length

(See Hemline.)

Sleeve

The portion of the wedding gown that covers the

arms. Some sleeve styles can be combined with others (e.g., bishop and illusion). The common sleeve types are bishop, dolman, fitted, gigot, Juliet, melon, poet, renaissance, tapered, and tulip. Sleeves can be on or off the shoulder. When off the shoulder, they are known as dropped sleeves. Sleeves are usually made with the same fabric as the bodice, but can also be made with illusion to soften their effect.

Sleeve Lengths

Sleeve length terms are based on where the sleeve falls on the bride's arm. The common sleeve lengths are:

Cap: A very short sleeve only covering the shoulder. Also known by the names cap fitted and capped. A wide halter strap placed on the shoulder can be described as a cap sleeve length. Best suited for slender or well-toned upper arms.

Short: Falling midway between shoulder and elbow (longer than cap).

Elbow: A sleeve that extends to the elbow.

Three-Quarter: A sleeve that ends midway between the elbow and the wrist; this sleeve can make short arms appear longer.

Long: A sleeve that extends to the wrist.

Snood

Netting that holds the bride's hair at the nape of the neck.

Spaghetti Straps

A thin tubular strap that attaches to the bodice. Named for its likeness to a strand of spaghetti.

Spaghetti straps can be used to replace traditional shoulder straps for most necklines. When combined with scoop, square, or sweetheart necklines, the resulting bodice is known as a ballerina bodice.

Specified Neckline

A specified neckline refers to a particular type of neckline. For example, a V-neck is a specific style of neckline.

Split Neckline

(See Notched-V.)

Spray

Sometimes called a side spray, these headpieces usually do not have any veiling. They are often loose clusters of flowers and beading.

Square Neckline

A neckline that forms the outline of a square. On a strapless gown, a square neckline consists of a straight line across the top of the bodice.

Straight Cuff

Any cuff with a straight and uniform edge at the hem.

Straight Silhouette

(See Column Silhouette.)

Straight Skirt

(See Column Skirt.)

Straight Sleeve

This is the sleeve usually found on women's and

men's shirts. It can be used with or without a band at the cuff.

Straight Waist

(1) A waist design that is basic and unadorned.

(2) A simple seam or band around the waist to highlight the waist.

Strapless Bodice

A corseted bodice with no straps. The corset may or may not be incorporated into the exterior design of the bodice. (See Corseted Bodice.)

Strapless Neckline

A compound neckline created by combining a scoop, square, or sweetheart neckline with a strapless and sleeveless bodice.

Straps

Fabric used to carry (hold up) the bodice. Strap width and style can also affect the perceived width of a bride's shoulders. (See Spaghetti Straps and Halters.)

Stretch Brocade

(See Brocade.)

Sweetheart Neckline

A graceful neckline shaped like the top half of a heart over the bosom.

T-Style Necklace

A princess (hanging strand) necklace with a dangling strand hanging down from the bottom of the necklace, generally forming a "T" design.

Taffeta

A crisp, plain-woven lustrous fabric of various fibers used especially for women's clothing.

Tank Dress

A sleeveless form of a tent dress.

Tank Top Neckline

A compound neckline created by combining a scoop neckline with a sleeveless, usually fitted bodice.

Tapered Cuff

(See Pointed Cuff.)

Tapered Sleeve

Full from the shoulder to the elbow, then fitted to the wrist. Similar to a bishop sleeve, but not as full.

Tent Dress

A long, full dress that falls in a straight line from the shoulders to the ankles and does not follow the curves of the body.

Three-Quarter Glove

This is a six- or eight-button length glove that measures from the tip of the middle finger to a point two to four inches below the elbow. This glove is also known as a coat length glove. These gloves are the most versatile and can be used with any sleeve length. When used with the longer sleeves (three-quarter or long sleeves), they should be tucked under the sleeve.

GLOSSARY

Three-Quarter Sleeve

(See Sleeve Lengths.)

Tiara Headpiece

A decorative jeweled or flowered, circular headpiece. It is usually thin or open at the back, broadening as it comes around the head, and finally peaking over the forehead. Generally, tiaras are smaller than crowns. They are often used with a veil.

Tiered Skirt

A skirt built up of layered cloth. (See also Peplum.)

Tiered Train

(See Peplum.)

Tiered Veil

(See Cascade Veil.)

Traditional Bridal Look

Deals with customs and/or religious practices involved in a wedding. For example, it is traditional for a first time bride to wear white. (See Classic Bridal Look and Modern Bridal Look.)

Traditional Silhouette

(See Ball Silhouette.)

Train

The portion of a wedding gown that trails on the floor behind the bride. Trains can be elongated from the back hemline of the gown or attached at the waist or hips. One unique form, the watteau train, hangs from the shoulders. A fishtail train is narrow at the waist and flares dramatically at the knees in a fishtail shape.

Train Length

Tradition has given names to trains of varying lengths. Lengths are measured from the rear hem of the gown at floor length. Some names are used interchangeably; therefore, brides should confirm the actual length of their train with their dressmaker. Common train names are:

Sweep: Measured 8"–12" from a floor-length skirt hem. Also known as floor, duster, and brush trains.

Court: Measured 12"–36" from a floor-length skirt hem.

Chapel: Measured 36"–48" from a floor-length skirt hem. Also known as a medium train. This is the most popular train length.

Semi-cathedral: Measured 48"–72" from a floor-length skirt hem.

Cathedral: Measured 72"–96" from a floor-length skirt hem. This train is usually reserved for formal weddings.

Royal Cathedral: Measured 96"–120" from a floor-length skirt hem. Also known as a traditional royal train. This train is usually reserved for formal weddings.

Monarch: Measured 144" or more from a floor-length skirt hem. Also known as a royal train. This train is usually reserved for the most formal weddings.

Trumpet Skirt

A slim, body-hugging skirt that flares out beginning mid-thigh. A trumpet skirt is the centerpiece of the mermaid silhouette.

Tulip Sleeve

A cap sleeve made of overlapping fabric that curves into a petal-like shape over the top of the arm.

Tulle Skirt

(See Bouffant Skirt.)

U-Basque Waist

(See Curved Basque Waist.)

V-Band Headpiece

A type of halo headpiece that is placed low on the forehead and has a distinctive V-shaped dip over the eyes.

V-Neck Neckline

A neckline coming to a "V" shape over the bosom.

V-Waist

(See Basque Waist.)

Veil

A length of cloth worn by brides as a covering for the head and shoulders and often for the face. Veils are usually made with a foundation of veil illusion and then a veil design. Tradition has given names to veils of varying lengths. No specific length defines any given name as many are measured to various locations on the bride's body. Lengths are measured from the crown of the head. Some names are used interchangeably, brides should therefore confirm the actual length of their veil with their dressmaker. Veils are often referred to by a combination of length and style name; for example, "fingertip cascade veil" or "chapel-length back veil." The following are common names by length:

Shoulder: Measured to the shoulders (18"– 24").

Elbow/Waist: Measured to the elbows or waist (24"–38"). The distances to your elbows and waist can vary by several inches, but they both fit within the range of this one measurement. Whether you choose one over the other depends on how much the two distances vary.

Fingertip: Measured to the tips of the index fingers when the arms are allowed to hang loose (38"–40").

Knee: Measured to the knees (40"–50").

Ballet (Waltz): Measured to the mid-point between the knees and ankles (50"–60"). Also known as a ballerina veil.

Sweep: Measured to the floor (60"–72").

Chapel: Veil falls behind the bride by two or three feet (72"–90").

Cathedral: Veil falls behind the bride by three to five feet (108"–140"). Veil may be attached at the crown of the head, at the shoulders, or at the waist.

Royal Cathedral: Veil falls behind the bride by five to eight feet (140"–180"). Also known as a regal or monarch veil. This veil is often connected at the shoulders or waist due to its weight, and combined with a fingertip or waist veil to create a cascade.

Veil Design

Refers to the edging and accents used on veil illusion to produce a finished effect. Common styles are: plain edge, lettuce edge, pencil edge, satin cord, ribbon edge, lace edge, embroidered edge, nylon filament edge, pearl edge, pearl zig-zag edge, pearl scattered, sequin scattered, pearl galaxy, rhinestone edge, rhinestone scattered, and motif scattered.

Veil Illusion

Sheer veil fabric (see Illusion), commonly constructed of a fine tulle or other netting in the following colors: white, ivory, diamond white (an off-white), sparkle white, or sparkle ivory. Veil illusion can be ornamented with lace, embroidery, jewels, pearls, or appliqués.

Veil Shapes

How a veil lies and how it covers the body is determined by the cut of the veil.

Diamond: Starts at a point on the head, flares dramatically around the mid-point tapering to a point at the end.

Oval: Starts at a point on the head, flares gently around the mid-point tapering to a rounded end.

Square: With or without rounded corners, surrounds the head with a uniform flare to the end.

Velvet

A clothing and upholstery fabric (as of silk, ray-on, or wool) characterized by a short, soft, dense warp pile.

Waist

The transition between the bodice and the skirt. The common waist styles are asymmetrical, basque, inverted-V, plain, shirred, and straight.

Waist Height

The waistline of a gown is not necessarily at the body's waist. A gown's waist can be adjusted for both effect and to compensate for body shape. There are four standard waist heights: dropped, natural, raised, and empire.

Watteau Train

A train attached at the shoulders rather than an elongation of the rear hem of the gown. A cathedral (or larger) veil worn with a gown having no train is said to be a watteau train. (Also known as a capelet train.)

Wedding Band Neckline

This is a formal, very high collar that fits snugly around the middle of the neck and just brushes the chin in a choker effect. It can be ornate or plain, and frequently tops a lace or net overlay that reveals portions of the upper chest. It is also known as a high collar neckline. The Queen Anne and Queen Elizabeth necklines are variations of the wedding band neckline.

Wide Cuff

A cuff that incorporates a wide, fitted band of material. Considered in the extreme, a Juliet sleeve uses a wide cuff that extends from the wrist to above the elbow.

Wreath Headpiece

A garland or ring of flowers encircling the head. Can be used with or without a veil. (See Halo Headpiece.)

Wrist Glove

This is the shortest of the gloves. It generally measures from the tip of the middle finger to near or at the wrist.

Photograph Acknowledgments

Photograph descriptions come from the manufacturer and may not use the definitions provided in this book. See the Acknowledgments section on page xv for manufacturer contact information.

Stock photography on the following pages provided by iStockphoto.com: i, iii, 40–41, 50, 60, 65, 66–67, 69, 83–84, 86–88, 94–95, 102–105, 108–109, 112–114, 120–121

Cover Style #1231, net over satin, crystal beading, sequins, re-embroidered lace, strapless princess line dress with chapel train, courtesy Alfred Angelo.

Cover Style #1505, satin, chiffon over satin embroidery, crystal and pearl beading, sequins, princess line dress with strapless bodice and empire waistline, courtesy Alfred Angelo.

Cover Style #9E8787, satin floor-length halter gown with cascading side drape and flower detail, courtesy David's Bridal.

xi   Courtesy Olga Ramos, Model

xiii   Courtesy Kathleen Bennett, Model

xiii   Courtesy Nelle Gilbert, Model

xiii   Courtesy Terreece Clarke, Model

xx   Style #AP6030, Aurora Formals collection, organza/netting, shawl and 1" detachable straps included, courtesy The Formal Source.

1   Courtesy Chenese Lewis, Miss Plus America 2003.

3   Style #ADP7400, Aurora D'Paradiso collection, spun gold floral beaded matte satin faux two piece odice with organza skirt, chapel train, satin edged organza shawl included, courtesy The Formal Source.

7   Style #6826, Aurora D'Paradiso collection, matte satin, laser-burnout lace with glass beads, seed pearls, and sequins, cathedral train, courtesy The Formal Source

8   Style #1231, net over satin, crystal beading, sequins, re-embroidered lace, strapless princess line dress with chapel train, courtesy Alfred Angelo.

9   Courtesy Peggy Lutz Plus.

9   Style #1505, satin, chiffon over satin embroidery, crystal and pearl beading, sequins, princess line dress with strapless bodice and empire waistline, courtesy Alfred Angelo.

10   Style #1963, taffeta embroidery, crystal beading, sequins with semi-cathedral train, courtesy Alfred Angelo.

10   Style #1202, net over satin, re-embroidered

lace, beading, strapless with flare gown, net shawl with matching lace and beading, with chapel train, courtesy Alfred Angelo.

10   Style #3281, Aurora D'Paradiso collection, beaded venise lace, matte satin / organza with detachable train, courtesy The Formal Source.

10   Style #9003A, beaded lace sheath with pearl halter neckline and detachable chiffon back panel, courtesy David's Bridal.

11   Style #6282 courtesy The Formal Source

12   Style #7427, Aurora D'Paradiso collection, directly beaded matte satin, cathedral train, courtesy The Formal Source.

13   Courtesy Rose Maloney.

14   Style #7416 courtesy The Formal Source

14   Style #5024, Aurora D'Paradiso collection, beaded illusion, matte satin, courtesy The Formal Source.

14   Style #7426, Aurora D'Paradiso collection, beaded english netting over matte satin, cathedral train, courtesy The Formal Source.

14   Style #9S8455 courtesy David's Bridal

15   Style #1945, luster satin, re-embroidered metallic lace, crystal beading, sequins, sweetheart neckline with asymmetric drape, a-line gown, satin covered buttons, semi-cathedral train, courtesy Alfred Angelo.

15   Style #7415 courtesy The Formal Source.

16   Style #6835, Aurora D'Paradiso collection,

matte satin, 1" detachable straps & removable modesty panel, cathedral train, courtesy The Formal Source.

16   Style #6826, Aurora D'Paradiso collection, matte satin, laser-burnout lace with glass beads, seed pearls, and sequins, cathedral train, courtesy The Formal Source

17   Style #5024, Aurora D'Paradiso collection, beaded illusion, matte satin, courtesy The Formal Source.

17   Style #24222, courtesy Mon Cheri Bridals.

18   Style #9T8077, chiffon split-front empire a-line with beaded lace trim, sweep train, available in ivory or white, courtesy David's Bridal.

19   Courtesy Peggy Lutz Plus.

19   Style #5031, courtesy The Formal Source.

19   Style #9N8579, satin v-neck halter gown with beading on the bodice, courtesy David's Bridal.

21   Style #7401, Aurora D'Paradiso collection, embroidery accented with ice blue highlights on netting, chapel train, courtesy The Formal Source.

22   Style #9S8455 courtesy David's Bridal

22   Style #9003A, beaded lace sheath with pearl halter neckline and detachable chiffon back panel, courtesy David's Bridal

23   Courtesy Peggy Lutz Plus.

23   Style #7425, Aurora D'Paradiso collection, directly beaded matte satin bodice with chif-

ACKNOWLEDGMENTS

fon skirt, chapel train, chiffon shawl included, courtesy The Formal Source.

24   Style #1945, luster satin, re-embroidered metallic lace, crystal beading, sequins, sweetheart neckline with asymmetric drape, a-line gown, satin covered buttons, semi-cathedral train, courtesy Alfred Angelo.

25   Style #98570, satin floor-length gown with off-the-shoulder portrait collar and back bow detail, courtesy David's Bridal.

25   Style #5053, Aurora D'Paradiso collection, directly beaded soft duchess satin, cathedral train, courtesy The Formal Source.

25   Style #9N8579, satin v-neck halter gown with beading on the bodice, courtesy David's Bridal.

26   Style #4178, Aurora D'Paradiso collection, bugle bead trimmed chiffon, courtesy The Formal Source.

26   Style #9T8076, strapless satin a-line gown with side-draped bodice and asymmetric skirt, courtesy David's Bridal.

27   Style #9E8052, strapless satin a-line with lace-up back and sweep train, available with a variety of color trims, courtesy David's Bridal.

28   Style #98570, satin floor-length gown with off-the-shoulder portrait collar and back bow detail, courtesy David's Bridal.

28   Style #2352, courtesy The Formal Source.

28   Courtesy Rose Mahoney

29   Style #4178, Aurora D'Paradiso collection, bugle bead trimmed chiffon, courtesy The Formal Source.

29   Style #7409, Aurora D'Paradiso collection, chiffon floor length gown with austrian crystals, bugle beads and sequins, removable tank chiffon coat chapel train, courtesy The Formal Source.

29   Style #91110, courtesy David's Bridal.

29   Style #3278, Aurora D'Paradiso collection, embroidered chiffon, courtesy The Formal Source.

29   Courtesy Peggy Lutz Plus.

30   Style #4167, Aurora D'Paradiso collection, bead accented corded lace, matte satin, courtesy The Formal Source.

30   Style #5025, courtesy The Formal Source.

30   Style #98570, satin floor-length gown with off-the-shoulder portrait collar and back bow detail, courtesy David's Bridal.

30   Style #4177, Aurora D'Paradiso collection, beaded embroidery, matte satin, courtesy The Formal Source.

31   Style #9T8076, strapless satin a-line gown with side-draped bodice and asymmetric skirt, courtesy David's Bridal.

31   Style #9V8377, courtesy David's Bridal.

32   Single silver edge flyaway veil, courtesy All You Need is Love.

34   Custom and hand-made 45" fingertip length oval cut veil with 35" top tier trimmed with

an embroidered edge and scattered pearls, courtesy Veil Artistry.

34 Custom and hand-made 60" diamond cut veil with 5/8" satin ribbon edge, courtesy Veil Artistry.

34 Custom and hand-made 45" fingertip length square cut veil with scattered Swarovski® crystal clusters, courtesy Veil Artistry.

35 Style #9E8052, strapless satin a-line with lace-up back and sweep train, available with a variety of color trims, courtesy David's Bridal.

36 Style #9E8787, satin floor-length halter gown with cascading side drape and flower detail, courtesy David's Bridal.

37 Custom and hand-made 45" angel veil trimmed with 3/8" sheer organza ribbon, courtesy Veil Artistry.

37 Custom and hand-made 72" back veil with modified butterfly cut, courtesy Veil Artistry.

38 Custom and hand-made birdcage veil attached to a pillbox hat, courtesy Veil Artistry.

38 Custom and hand-made 22" butterfly veil accented with floral embroidery, courtesy Veil Artistry.

38 Custom and hand-made 18" flyaway veil trimmed with 1/4" satin ribbon, courtesy Veil Artistry.

38 Custom and hand-made 24" fountain veil (16" top tier) trimmed with bias-bound satin fabric, courtesy Veil Artistry.

38 Custom and hand-made 30" mantilla veil trimmed with 2-3/8" cluny lace, courtesy Veil Artistry.

39 Custom and hand-made "cloud" pouf veil attached to a v-band pearl halo, courtesy Veil Artistry.

39 Style #9E8561, strapless organza gown featuring a side drape, shirring scattered beadings and a chapel train, courtesy David's Bridal.

40 Custom hand-made Swarovski® crystal bun ring with 6mm and 4mm aurora borealis crystals, courtesy Veil Artistry.

40 Custom hand-made satin teardrop cap embellished with alencon lace, pearls, and sequins courtesy Veil Artistry.

40 Custom hand-made jeweled comb featuring Swarovski® marquis rhinestone, round, and floral crystals courtesy Veil Artistry.

40 Custom crafted 1-1/4" crown embellished with sparkling glass crystals courtesy Veil Artistry.

41 Custom hand-made v-band halo made from satin cording and 3mm pearls, courtesy Veil Artistry.

41 Custom crafted headband made with 4mm Swarovski® clear bicone crystals, courtesy Veil Artistry.

41 Custom hand-made spray headpiece featuring ivory tiger lily, courtesy Veil Artistry.

41 Custom hand-made 1-1/4" center-measure tiara embellished with 8mm, 6mm, and 4mm

ACKNOWLEDGMENTS

Swarovski® round faceted clear and amethyst crystals courtesy, Veil Artistry.

43 Courtesy Peggy Lutz Plus.

43 Courtesy Peggy Lutz Plus.

43 Style #1231, net over satin, crystal beading, sequins, re-embroidered lace, strapless princess line dress with chapel train, courtesy Alfred Angelo.

43 Style #1774, re-embroidered lace on net, pearl and crystal beading, strapless neckline, dropped waist, high-low hemline, removable satin skirt with chapel train, courtesy Alfred Angelo.

44 Style #6834, Aurora D'Paradiso collection, matte satin, organza carriage, chapel train, courtesy The Formal Source.

44 Style #2320, Aurora D'Paradiso collection, beaded allencon lace, matte satin, courtesy The Formal Source.

44 Style #1425, satin, metallic embroidery, crystal beading, sequins, trumpet skirt, covered buttons back detail, optional spaghetti straps included, chapel train, courtesy Alfred Angelo.

45 Style #1488, tulle over satin, tulle, sequins, embroidery crystal beading, courtesy Alfred Angelo.

45 Style #7425, Aurora D'Paradiso collection, directly beaded matte satin bodice with chiffon skirt, chapel train, chiffon shawl included, courtesy The Formal Source.

46 Style #1202, net over satin, re-embroidered lace, beading, strapless with flare gown, net shawl with matching lace and beading with chapel train courtesy Alfred Angelo.

46 Style #1963, taffeta embroidery, crystal beading, sequins with semi-cathedral train, courtesy Alfred Angelo.

46 Style #7406, Aurora D'Paradiso collection, matte satin encrusted with austrian crystals, pearls and glass beads, chapel train, courtesy The Formal Source.

46 Style #2380, Aurora D'Paradiso collection, directly beaded organza, 1" detachable beaded straps chapel train, courtesy The Formal Source.

46 Style #2380, Aurora D'Paradiso collection, directly beaded organza, 1" detachable beaded straps chapel train, courtesy The Formal Source.

46 Style #1202, net over satin, re-embroidered lace, beading, strapless with flare gown, net shawl with matching lace and beading with chapel train, courtesy Alfred Angelo.

48 Style #9E8052, strapless satin a-line with lace-up back and sweep train, available with a variety of color trims, courtesy David's Bridal.

48 Courtesy Ramona Keveza.

48 Style #9T8640, satin ball gown adorned with beaded lace features back button detailing and cathedral train with cut-out lace appliques, courtesy David's Bridal.

48 Style #95268, embroidered satin a-line with

split front overskirt, courtesy David's Bridal.

49   Courtesy Peggy Lutz Plus.

49   Courtesy Peggy Lutz Plus.

49   Courtesy Peggy Lutz Plus.

49   Courtesy Peggy Lutz Plus.

49   Style #9003A, beaded lace sheath with pearl halter neckline and detachable chiffon back panel, courtesy David's Bridal.

54   Style #C600323, bridal charmeuse and lace, courtesy About Curves.

54   Style #BU6709, wedding wishes corset, courtesy About Curves.

57   Courtesy Cori Photography.

57   Style #5051, courtesy The Formal Source.

58   Style #6386, courtesy The Formal Source.

59   Courtesy Peggy Lutz Plus.

59   Courtesy Cynthia Woodlief, model.

61   Courtesy Peggy Lutz Plus.

62   Style #2379, Aurora D'Paradiso collection, directly beaded matte satin, 1" detachable straps chapel train, courtesy The Formal Source.

71   Courtesy Chamein Canton, author.

75   Courtesy Charissa Sylvester, model

75   Courtesy Olga Ramos, model.

75   Style #9003A, beaded lace sheath with pearl halter neckline and detachable chiffon back panel, courtesy David's Bridal.

75   Style #5051, courtesy The Formal Source.

76   Courtesy Cynthia Woodlief, model.

76   Style #1243, satin, crystal beading, pearls, rhinestones, two-piece look, strapless bodice with scalloped neckline, a-line skirt with double layer apron back, optional beaded straps, semi-cathedral train, courtesy Alfred Angelo.

76   Style #9T8076, strapless satin a-line gown with side-draped bodice and asymmetric skirt, courtesy David's Bridal.

80   Courtesy Terreece Clarke, model.

93   Courtesy Peggy Lutz Plus.

101   Style #7416, Aurora D'Paradiso collection, courtesy The Formal Source.

106   Courtesy Peggy Lutz Plus.

107   Style #5022, Aurora Formals collection, iridescent satin, plain iridescent satin shawl included, courtesy The Formal Source.

111   Courtesy Debra A. Hawks, model.

111   Courtesy Rose Maloney, model.

111   Courtesy Debra A. Hawks, model.

111   Courtesy Courtesy Peggy Lutz Plus.

111   Style #1505, satin, chiffon over satin embroidery, crystal and pearl beading, sequins, princess line dress with strapless bodice and empire waistline. courtesy Alfred Angelo.

ACKNOWLEDGMENTS

117   Courtesy Madame Butterfly Cakes.

118   Courtesy Cori Photography.

124   Style #7408, Aurora Formals collection, matte satin, embroidery accented with austrian crystals, pearls, sequins and glass beads, chapel train, pearl trimmed chiffon bolero, courtesy The Formal Source.

127   Courtesy Chamein Canton, author.

Back Cover Photos:

Courtesy Kelli Herbert, model.

Courtesy Charissa Sylvester, model.

Courtesy The Formal Source.

Index

INDEX

INDEX